Patient Safety in Clinical]

This book introduces the core knowledge and skills for comprehensive risk assessment and management in healthcare settings and applies relevant ethical and legal principles. It emphasises that patient safety requires a holistic and inclusive approach to maximise patient wellbeing in a diverse population with known health inequalities.

Exploring the concept of 'avoidable risks' which may be posed to the health and wellbeing of individuals, the public and communities within a given healthcare context, this book explores potential system failures and human factors, while providing an insight into the significance of the relationship between a culture of care and patient safety. It includes chapters on the ethical and legal framework related to patient safety, the equality, diversity and inclusion context, advocacy and empowerment, risk, and human factors as well as accountability and harm. Notably, there is also a focus on two in-depth chapters which explore patient safety in relation to medication management and end-of-life care.

Throughout the book, there are numerous reflection points, examples of case law and illustrative case studies and thinking points to help the reader apply key principles to aid their learning and think critically. *Patient Safety in Clinical Practice* offers a fresh insight into the link between patient safety and holistic care. It is aimed at nursing and allied health students and professionals, particularly those undertaking study related to assessing and planning care, as well as law, ethics and professional issues.

Paul Buka, MSc, PGCE, LLB (Hons) Law, HNC, RGN, RNT, FHEA, MIHSCM, Member of the Institute of Medical Ethics, is a visiting lecturer at the University of Essex. He specialises in Healthcare Law and Ethics, with several publications (since 1999) and a third edition book in 2020 to his name. He trained as a Registered General Nurse in Scotland, specialising in Trauma and Orthopaedics nursing, with many years of varied clinical experience. He read law at HNC, degree and master's levels, specialising in Criminal Justice, Human Rights, Clinical Negligence and Mental Health Law, and has working knowledge and experience of Health and Safety law and as a (Union) health and safety representative in Clinical Practice and HE. He gained 24 years of experience in Further Education and Higher Education as a former Programme Lead (senior lecturer). He served as a lay member for the Department of Health Regional Advisory Committee on Clinical Excellence Awards (ACCEA) for seven years.

"This is a well-written book, suitable for students and qualified healthcare professionals who wish to enhance their knowledge and understanding of patient safety. Complexities of law and ethics linked to patient safety are explored in a way that readers will easily understand, I strongly recommend it".
Ganapathy Ganesalingam, *RGN, BSc, PG Dip, MSc, Senior Lecturer in Adult Nursing, University of Greenwich*

"Safety is paramount in all aspects of a patient's journey as they engage with services, in hospital or community settings. The book explores patient safety, risk management and applies relevant ethical, and legal principles. I strongly recommend it for students, professionals in all areas of healthcare practice and research".
Dr Stephen Joseph, *BEd, MBA, RN, RMHN, MNSc, PgDMHN, PhD, Lecturer (Researcher) MH, University of Essex*

"Patient safety is the most fundamental aspect of healthcare and often it's marginalised groups and individuals who experience poorer outcomes and are exposed to more risks in clinical practice. Therefore, I recommend this book to all students and healthcare professionals to reflect on the content in this book, so we can work towards minimising risk in all clinical environments".
Dr Andrew Clifton, *PhD, MRes, PgDipLTHE, BA (Hons), RN (MH), FHEA, Associate Professor of Nursing, University of Suffolk*

"With a focus on ethical and legal foundations of promoting a safety culture in health and social care, this text is invaluable for professionals, staff and students entrusted with protecting vulnerable people in service provision settings. Using legal, bioethical, and clinical case scenarios to illustrate discussions, and thinking points to encourage personal reflection, issues are raised and explored in an accessible and considered way throughout".
Jim Sumpter, *Former lecturer, RN, MSc Nursing, Post-graduate Certificate in Inter-professional Education, University of Essex*

Patient Safety in Clinical Practice

A Diverse Approach to Safe Healthcare for All

Edited by Paul Buka

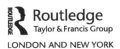

LONDON AND NEW YORK

Designed cover image: Shutterstock

First published 2025
by Routledge
4 Park Square, Milton Park, Abingdon, Oxon OX14 4RN

and by Routledge
605 Third Avenue, New York, NY 10158

Routledge is an imprint of the Taylor & Francis Group, an informa business

British Library Cataloguing-in-Publication Data
A catalogue record for this book is available from the British Library

ISBN: 978-1-032-45424-5 (hbk)
ISBN: 978-1-032-45423-8 (pbk)
ISBN: 978-1-003-37693-4 (ebk)

DOI: 10.4324/9781003376934

Typeset in Times New Roman
by KnowledgeWorks Global Ltd.

Dedication

To my wife Carol, for keeping me on track, my son, Alexander, his other half, Alannah and our awesome grandchildren, Joshua and Hana, and to their uncle – my son George. Thank you all for the reassurance and for putting up with me. Not forgetting, my in-laws, Laura and Jimmy for your encouragement as usual.

Contents

List of boxes

Preface

This project emerged over time, informed by the contributing authors' academic, clinical backgrounds, expertise, interests and their passion for 'patient safety', as applied to a variety of healthcare settings. There are currently a limited number of texts relevant to patient safety on the market, which are intended for healthcare professionals other than medical clinicians. The contributing authors aim to address key concepts which may impact a service user's safety and wellbeing and to do no harm. The focal context is one of 'holistic' and 'person-centred' care. The key consideration for healthcare delivery should be maximising the physical and/or psychological safety as well as the well-being while minimising the risk of harm to all.

The focal concept of 'patient safety' will be explored, subject to health and safety legislation, critically, the Health and Safety Act 1974 subordinate legislation and professional regulation, along with the intersection between the ethical and legal frameworks. The employer and employee both have a duty of care in Bioethics and Tort [Delict (Scots law)] to ensure the safety of patients, that of others as well as their own. The duty of care (above) on the part of the healthcare professional is a legal, ethical and professional requirement. Patients' and the staff's health and safety may be adversely affected due to unsafe or inappropriate actions or omissions. Subject to the above-mentioned United Kingdom health and safety legislative framework, all staff are also required to carry out risk assessments and to implement risk management plans to promote patients' safety, and that of others, including themselves.

Throughout the discourse, the terms 'patient' and 'service user' will be used interchangeably in accordance with national and professional bodies' guidance. Relevant terms not included here, such as 'customer', 'stakeholder' or 'client' may nevertheless be found in other related literature.

Marginalised groups in societies and communities are acknowledged in this text, as they are more likely to experience limited access to healthcare. This may be due to factors such as deprivation, limited access to healthcare or possible discrimination, resulting in poorer outcomes during their (marginalised groups') lifespan as they face health challenges. The focus here is on 'risk minimisation', 'hazards' and 'avoidable harm' while addressing health and safety concerns. The debate will be via the medium of equality, diversity and inclusion. Safety shortcomings can lead to an increased risk of physical and/or psychological harm for marginalised and vulnerable groups. The association between health inequalities and patient safety is inevitable and can be complex. An inclusive approach to safe care delivery is essential and should be at the focal point. Healthcare professionals should be guided by the law, Bioethics and, crucially, their own code of professional conduct.

Patients' safety concerns may have recently been exacerbated by the COVID-19 pandemic. This book encourages readers (managing clinical tasks) to engage in proactive assessment and management and minimise risk with an insight into the link between patient-centred and holistic care to achieve patient safety.

Within the discipline of Ethics or Moral Philosophy, the term 'Bioethics' is generic and much broader than Biomedical Ethics (or Principlism). This is because Bioethics derives from the application of Classical Ethical theories to multiple disciplines related to social policy. Examples are in business, legal and healthcare professions. Bioethics is regarded as 'equivalent to medical ethics, or biomedical ethics' Britannica (no date). Biomedical Ethics or Bioethics plays a key part in shaping the focus on the 'To do no harm' principle in the context of the law and its relationship with professional regulation. 'Bioethics' is the preferred term which will be used in this book. Any caring relationship should be 'fiduciary', i.e., based on trust. Clinicians must work in partnership with and empower the service user while advocating for them a 'culture of care' and concordance. Bioethics informs the law and regulates citizens' and healthcare professionals' conduct. Although key aspects of the law herein are based on United Kingdom law, this may be applicable to comparable international legal systems which are 'Common Law'-based, as well as Roman-Dutch Law systems. The authors recognise the need, wherever practicable, for every effort to be made to highlight any key distinctions in UK law subject to application to Scotland and Northern Ireland. Due to the limited nature and size of this book, a comprehensive and detailed analysis is not practicable, and any specific reference will be only made as necessary. The UK legal context will normally be incorporated and applied.

As potential system failures or human factors are identified, greater awareness of equality, diversity and inclusion will inform a more comprehensive approach. Clinicians should also learn not only from when something went wrong but also when all goes according to plan. Harm or near misses may result from systemic failures and/or human errors. The onus on individual healthcare professionals is to raise concerns on potential or actual risks and to safeguard and whistleblow to ensure that patients or service users are not exposed to the risk of harm.

The authors have in mind final-year degree and CPD students for nursing (all branches). Multi-disciplinary students and healthcare professionals will also find this book useful. Qualified healthcare professionals may also benefit from the content as a basis for reflection.

Contributing authors will incorporate different learning modalities, for engaging readers with differing learning styles. Relevant perspectives will be addressed while encouraging reflection. This includes case law, case studies/scenarios and thinking points to aid the reader's 'questioning mind', learning and/or curiosity.

This should encourage students and healthcare professionals to enhance their clinical and leadership skills and to think reflectively and critically, with a questioning mind, to assess, manage as well as minimise risk for all (including themselves) within a healthcare environment.

Finally, the authors draw on their individual academic knowledge and varied clinical experiences, applying theory and reflecting on real-life clinical practice case scenarios while maintaining confidentiality, real case studies (in the public domain) case scenarios, as well as cited case law.

References

Britannica (no date) https://www.britannica.com/topic/bioethics
Health and Safety at Work Act (1974) https://www.hse.gov.uk/legislation/hswa.htm

Foreword

It is an immense privilege and honour to be invited to write the foreword to a book that resonates so much with contemporary safe professional practice, with the patient at the heart of all we do.

Patient Safety in Clinical Practice offers an analytical approach to understanding the legal and ethical issues of concern, and practical application and evaluation of the conceptual frameworks that inform patient safety systems. In their daily practice, health and social care professionals are confronted with challenges that test their abilities to make rational and ethical decisions, which have an impact on achieving the best outcomes for patients. Healthcare challenges are complex, multidimensional and involve professional working in systems governing quality and safety. This involves working with others. Healthcare practitioners may be held to account for actions, and omissions, where a patient may have been harmed or at risk. Healthcare systems may experience resources constraints, manpower issues and increasing demands, resulting in varied quality of care affecting patient safety.

Understanding and applying legal and ethical principles and adherence to guidelines in clinical practice ensure that providers' aim to achieve patient safety to the standards set out in professional regulations and statutes can be realised. Adopting an inclusive approach, the authors have drawn from their vast experience in clinical practice and professional education to bring together the legal frameworks underpinning autonomous practice and clinical governance, the ethical concerns pertinent to the vulnerability of diverse patient groups and their safety. In their articulation of actual and recorded problems and outcomes, case studies have been selected to demonstrate relevance and evaluation, and policy-making and implications for the reduction of harm to patients. The severity of the outcomes can also be understood in the context of whichever practice settings and patient groups are being supported and treated. The areas of knowledge informing practice are drawn from a wide range of sources from law, ethics and medical and social sciences. Herein lies the strength of this book, offering critical academic and practical insights into complex human scenarios.

The patient's journey depends as much on the patient-associated factors as it does on the systems of care and encounters with different health and social care professionals. With populations becoming increasingly diverse in characteristics, equality and equity issues warrant consideration from the perspectives of culture, language, belief systems and abilities. As the subtitle suggests, 'A Diverse Approach to Safe Healthcare for All' is embedded in the exploration of health and care needs, the legal and ethical concerns, and utilisation methods and measure to avert potential risks and overcome conflicts. The ability and capacity of patients to communicate, consent to treatment and make informed decisions are predicated by healthcare professionals being aware and competent in dealing with situations ethically and exercising their skills in forming trusting and therapeutic interactions. Explanation of concepts associated with inequalities, diversity and justice and their significance to the pursuance of safe and high-standard care are addressed with clarity and in an engaging and pragmatic approach.

Patient safety holds a high priority in the agenda for care delivery in provider organisations. The book informs and guides policy analysis which is relevant to the exploration of the ethical and legal issues appropriate to varied settings and specialities. Where there are tensions between the legal and ethical frameworks, practice and professionalism, the reader is invited to reflect on triggers that capture the main propositions and arguments, thus allowing for debate and consolidation of the essence of safe practice. Personal responsibility, duty of care, leadership and culture of safety refocus the values and expectations of professional practice. With emerging new bioethical challenges in the age of increasing digitisation, e-health, unprecedented global health crises, disparities in healthcare and natural disasters, the health professional has much to reflect on and learn at every stage. This is from diagnosis to interventions, from recovery to end-of life to practice safely and ethically within the legal regulations. The reader, whatever their health profession, will find this book invaluable in supporting their learning and practice, in whichever settings they encounter patients and their families.

The authors have moulded the content to appeal to clinicians and non-clinicians, students undertaking a wide range of professional education programmes in medicine and allied health professions, administration, and ethics and law. Equally, it will be of interest to the lay person, patient organisations and international health workforce.

I recommend this book in the genuine belief that what I have read offers the reader unparalleled working insight into the legal and ethical issues applicable to practice and reinforcing patient safety as the key target outcome for professional practice.

Dave Sookhoo, RN, BA, MEd, PhD
Associate Lecturer, University of Sunderland
in London and Open University, UK

Biography

David Atkinson, MA, MEd, BSc, RN, FHEA, Member of the Institute for Medical Ethics, He is a Member of the International Forum of Teachers of the UNESCO Chair in Bioethics since 2016 and a Fellow of the Higher Education Academy since 2006. He is lecturer in Adult Nursing at the University of Suffolk, with over 20 years' experience and has worked at two other universities. He has an MA in Medical Ethics and Law and a master's degree in education and published in healthcare law and ethics. Areas of interest include Medical Ethics and Law and Leadership and Management.

Cheyne Truman, BSc (Hons) Adult, RN, FHEA, is lecturer in nursing at the University of Essex. She was a reviewer for the publication 'Essential law and ethics in nursing, patients' rights, and decision-making' (2020), third edition. She has also published several articles, blogs and opinion pieces in the Nursing Times from 2018 to 2023. Cheyne is a Registered Nurse specialising in end-of-life and palliative nursing care, having worked in acute oncology and respiratory care. Cheyne is currently working towards her Medical and Clinical Education postgraduate degree. Cheyne draws upon her experience exceeding 15 years within the healthcare sector working with vulnerable and elderly people in a range of settings. Cheyne is in her early academic career delivering higher education to nursing students on BSC and MSc pathways as well as apprenticeships. She draws upon experience nursing on the frontline during the COVID-19 pandemic caring for vulnerable people at the most critical times, including end-of-life. She also delivers nursing education with experience as an alumna of the University of Essex.

Acknowledgements

I am indebted to the staff at Routledge; Taylor & Francis, firstly, to Grace McInnes, Publisher, for her guidance and support, from start to finish, and also Madii Cherri-Moreton, Editorial Assistant, for the painstaking work and for patiently responding to my many emails. Thank you also to Riya and the production team at KGL whose hard work made this project possible. I am also much obliged to the 'co-authors', David Atkinson and Cheyne Truman, for their invaluable input, knowledge, experience and for sharing their individual expertise, I couldn't have made it without your valuable input.

On behalf of the contributing authors, we are all grateful to colleagues who kindly peer-reviewed drafts, as they tried to make sense of the chapters while providing invaluable feedback: Mr Ganapathy Ganesalingam, Senior Lecturer in Adult Nursing, University of Greenwich; Mrs Jenny Bacon, Ward Sister (In-Patients Unit), St Luke's Hospice, Essex; Dr Andrew Clifton, Associate Professor of Nursing, University of Suffolk; Mr Jim Sumpter, former lecturer in Adult Nursing, University of Essex; Dr Stephen Joseph, lecturer, University of Essex for the critical review and Mrs Laura Carlin, senior staff nurse (recently retired), Dundee, Scotland. We are also grateful to Dr Dave Sookhoo, University of Sutherland and Open University, for kindly doing the peer review of the project and for the brilliant and comprehensive foreword.

Thank you also to all academic colleagues and students past and present, who we are privileged to have known for their formal feedback and questioning minds. Finally, not forgetting the key player(s), patients or service users (anonymised), who I may have been privileged to meet or work with during my clinical practice and academic career.

1 Development of a patient safety culture

Paul Buka

Introduction

Safety is paramount in all healthcare settings and at the heart of planning care. The term 'patient' or 'service user' will be used interchangeably in this context. The relationship between clinicians and patients at all levels is fiduciary, which means that this is unequal and based on 'trust'. This means control by the clinician vis-à-vis dependence by the patient, which means a relationship seemingly in favour of the clinician. The Paternalistic Model expects patients to take on a passive role for patients, with *'(patients')* lives literary in their *(clinician's)* hands' (Geezer Retro, 2021). Paternalism was synonymous with blind 'trust' in doctors and other healthcare professionals such as nurses. This contrasts with Concordance, which is patient empowerment, and working in partnership, (NHS Constitution, 2012, 2019). The World Health Organization (2023) identifies key patient safety issues:

- Around 1 in every 10 patients is harmed in healthcare, and more than 3 million deaths occur annually due to unsafe care. In low- to middle-income countries, as many as 4 in 100 people die from unsafe care (1).
- Above 50% of harm (1 in every 20 patients) is preventable; half of this harm is attributed to medications (2,3).
- Some estimates suggest that as many as 4 in 10 patients are harmed in primary and ambulatory settings, while up to 80% (23.6–85%) of this harm can be avoided (4).

(WHO, 2023)

Aligned Bioethical principles and emerging themes will be developed below and addressed further in subsequent chapters. Clinical governance aimed at addressing safety in the UK, safety initiatives were introduced in the 1990s; this also saw the alignment of the Scottish Patient Safety Quality Improvement Programme as early as 2008. A recent framework is the NHS Patient Safety Strategy (2019, updated 2021). The discourse hereinafter and in subsequent chapters will follow the Common Law of England and Wales and Northern Ireland with a close alignment of the Roman Dutch Law which is related to Scots Law.

DOI: 10.4324/9781003376934-1

Ethical considerations and patients' safety

Ethical or moral considerations are relevant to human relations in healthcare. The emergence of Western Moral Philosophy or ethics goes as far back as classical civilisations, mainly Ancient Greek and Roman. Moral Philosophy is a foundation for this specialism and is more commonly known as 'Ethics'. The Nuremberg Trial exposed post-World War 2 in response to human rights abuses (in Nazi human experimentation). In the aftermath of the trials, human rights abuses were exposed in medical research. This saw the emergence of branches of ethics, the relevant one for healthcare being 'Bioethics'. There was a need to protect research participants, which should now be strictly followed and well documented and established in research ethics principles. Bioethics (Beauchamp and Childress, 2019) was grounded in the Greek Moral Philosophy schools of Socrates (384–322 BC), Plato (429–347 BC) and Aristotle (384–322 BC). Bioethics has been adopted by most healthcare regulatory bodies.

The ancient Babylonian empire and the reign of Hammurabi (1792–1750 BC) took significant steps towards safety awareness when treating people. This was the basis of the development of Codified laws in Moral Philosophy or Ethics. The ancient era was marked by harsh laws which were enacted with the aim of keeping 'order' and 'justice' for citizens. Such legislation had established exacting and harsh penalties for physicians who had made errors and harmed their patients as a result. Hammurabi's Code had aimed at protecting patients from harm, based on morality as it was seen at the time. Standard of care needed to be clearly defined to determine negligence or question of assessment of 'fault'. The Code was an extensive legal text. The Sumerian laws stipulated stringent and exacting laws (*lex talionis*) which determined the lives of citizens, i.e., the principle which demanded an 'eye for an eye', exacting punishment of the doctor or surgeon should the patient be harmed, as remedy. This was described as 'retributive justice'. Those who would find themselves on the receiving end could have included physicians who may have made an error or if a patient was harmed through human factors. One example is:

Code 218

If a physician performs an operation and kills someone or cuts out his eye, the doctor's hands shall be cut off.

> (https://extinctdoctorgood.com/2017/12/23/hammurabis-
> medical-regulation-code-1750-bc-noble-profession-
> has-always-been-regulated-cruelly/)

There would have been no margin for error permitted, and the code may have been seen as exacting and harsh and not necessarily considering human factors and the uncertainty of developing medical science as well as risk and unavoidable human factors.

The Greek classical code on medical ethics, better known as the Hippocratic Oath, embraced the four principles of ethics from Hippocrates, a Greek philosopher and physician (460–377 BC). Unlike this oath, Paternalism assumed that a physician knows what is best for patient under their care. Its approach seemed to be the basis for the outmoded relationship between physician and patient as applicable to recent 20th-century medicine. It could be argued that paternalism had been advocated with the aim to promote safety for patients 'in their best interests'. The General Medical Council guidance on patient safety is based on the 'To do no Harm' Principle as well as the Hippocratic Oath:

Domain 2. Safety and quality
Contribute to and comply with systems to protect patients.
Respond to risks to safety.
Protect patients and colleagues from any risk posed by your health (Good Medical
    Practice (GMC), 2019)
                    (https://patient.info/doctor/ideals-and-the-hippocratic-oath)

Ethics evolved from the classical moral frameworks from philosophers such as Socrates (470/469–399 BC) Plato (428/427–348/347 BC) and Aristotle (384–322 BC). In its broadest sense, ethics can be described as a system of rules or moral principles and often described as Bioethics or when (less commonly so, when applied to healthcare, as 'Biomedical Ethics' or 'Principlism'. The term 'Bioethics' is preferred.
    Bioethics focuses around:

- Respect for autonomy
- Beneficence
- Non maleficence
- Fairness or justice

The 'non-maleficence' will be the focal point of 'patient safety' (Beauchamp and Childress, 2019).
    Ethics is the precursor of law and may inform the latter. This is because where there is not always clear guidance, judges who apply the law may be guided by their own ethics or moral campus.

Emergence of hospitals, the historical context

The development of the first hospitals was linked to the Norman Conquest, in the aftermath of the Battle of Hasting 1066, the term 'hospital', which was derived from Latin for the word 'reception hospitium' for 'a guest', emerged. Some long-term beds were self-funded by the wealthy who would be guaranteed lifelong care. The healthcare system as we know it today took some time, with the NHS as the most significant development in 1948. This became synonymous with health for all 'from birth to death', the landmark of provision for a free service at the point of delivery. The concept of 'hospital' as mentioned above goes back much further in time. St Bartholomew Hospital (St Barts) was the precursor of 'hospitals' as we know them today and has now been part of the NHS since 1948. The National Health Service inception was from the NHS Act (1948) and NHS (Scotland) Act 1947.

St Barts was founded in 1123 by Rahere, who was a former courtier of Henry 1. This was probably the oldest hospital in the country though original buildings have now been replaced. Many of the so-called hospitals were in fact charitable almshouses for the poor and aged. Staffing for care and nursing was usually provided for by religious groups including monks and nuns. The overall standards were poor considering resources were few and far between. Infirmaries were originally built to look after elderly monks and nuns. Often there would be inevitable tension between clinicians and managers, '... there were reports of tensions between hospital managers and doctors as early as the 1700s, with doctors viewing the governors as suffocating and inefficient, and the governors regarding the doctors as their inferiors' (Sanai, 2006).

As early as the 18th century, people with mental health needs were admitted to institutions with the so-called criminally insane patients who also were deemed to have mental health needs. The so-called asylums were also associated with disease and poverty. These were crowded and poorly regulated institutions. The asylums were established and regulated by the County Asylums Act (1808). The first known one was opened as early as 1811, and the Lunacy (Scotland) Act 1857 pioneered mental health law. The care and treatment of residents was not good as indicated by the account of societal attitudes as shown below:

Did you know?

- Each county in the land was required to construct asylums to house people judged to be insane. Many counties failed to do this.
- Poet John Clare (1793–1864) spent 23 years in the St Andrew's Hospital in Northampton but was given freedom to wander round the town and local area.
- In some asylums 'it was the practice to chain patients by the leg, upon their first admission, in order to see what they would do'.
- The medical attendant at West Auckland Asylum considered that 'bleedings, blisters, and setons' were the principal resources of medicine for relieving 'maniacal excitement'.

(https://www.bbc.co.uk/history/familyhistory/bloodlines/
familysecrets.shtml?entry=county_asylum_
act&theme=familysecrets)

The Mental Health Act (1959) was the first legislative framework in England and Wales, following the Percy recommendations (1957). The statute clarified the distinction between mental health and other (general physical) hospitals by removing the confusion. This meant that those with mental health issues could be treated equally and benefit from general healthcare.

Subject to Section 6 (of the now repealed) Mental Health Act (1957), local authorities were required to provide aftercare in the community for those who did not require in patient care and:

1 providing and maintaining residential homes for people's care
2 providing and maintaining centres for training
3 providing ancillary or supplementary support services.
(https://navigator.health.org.uk/theme/mental-health-act-
1959#:~:text=The%20Act%20removed%20the%20distinction,
between%20mental%20and%20physical%20health)

The Mental Health Acts 1983 and 2007 are now the key statutes, providing for mental healthcare. Additionally, local authorities are required to provide adult social care in the community, under the Care Act (2014), in respect of needs at home or in residential care.

Safety in both physical and mental health hospitals had its own issues of the 'passive' patient versus the paternalistic clinician, however benevolent institutions may have intended. Service users may have been unaware of their rights, nor were they involved or active in decision-making then. They were usually grateful to receive benevolent care which they expected.

Human rights and patients' safety

The two world wars saw abuse and degradation of mainly Jewish prisoners of war as well as other vulnerable groups. There were serious breaches with inhuman experimentation in the name of medical research. The post-World War 2 Universal Declaration of Human Rights 1948 emerged from an international response aimed at defining and preservation of rights and prevention of future inhuman and degrading treatment of vulnerable people.

Thus, a foundation for human rights was laid in respect for all human beings and their safety as applied to safe delivery of health and social care, as provided by:

Article 3 of the European Convention on Human Rights (1950)

No one shall be subjected to torture or to inhuman or degrading treatment or punishment.

The statutory provision is in the European Convention of Human Rights Act 1950 (applied in the United Kingdom as the Human Rights Act, 1998). The legislation originated from the international treaty on the Universal Declaration of Human Rights, 1948). This defines a person's right not to be subjected to inhuman and degrading treatment.

In the United Kingdom, the concept of patient safety has evolved in time and goes as far back as the early 18th century. The development of Health and Safety legislation is linked to patient safety in the workplaces. This saw promotion of the safety of apprentices who were employed in the cotton mills and other factories. Progress was rather slow, much until the passing of the Factory Act 1802, which was supported by Sir Robert Peel (former prime minister) and subsequently adopted by the Church of England (Hurd, 2007).

An important milestone on safety in the workplace was reached when the Factory Acts 1833 and 1844 were passed. The latter statute aimed to consolidate the protection of children who were working in factories as apprentices. This was the most significant piece of legislation which became the remit of the HM Factories' Inspectorate with the enforcement of regulation. The Employers Liability Act (1969) (UK) was a significant milestone, in the right direction, towards safety. This was related to the protection of a worker who had been injured due to accidents caused by managers' actions. This statute applied to healthcare environments and made employers vicariously liable for the negligent actions of their employees.

Ethics as we have seen above are considered as the precursor and basis of law, and it also does inform the latter. This has also been applicable to employment law. This is because, where there is no clear guidance, judges may apply the law and they may be guided by their own ethics or moral campus. Ethical principles are broad and overlapping depending on the context. Before the Donoghue v Stevenson (1932, AC 562 HL) case (above), an ethics-based duty of care had been applied in establishing accountability, in a 19th-century negligence employment law case below:

Case Law: Priestley v Fowler [1837] 150 ER 1030

A claim was made by Priestly, the employee. This arose from the negligent decision of Thomas Fowler, the employer and defendant. This resulted in the claimant sustaining severe injuries following instructions to overload a wagon which subsequently overturned as a result, Thomas Fowler.

The claimant was awarded £100 damages.

The World Health Organization was founded post World War 2, in 1948 as a United Nations Agency and its policies, and to this day it has become the international cornerstone for defining and promoting safe practice and delivery of care for service users. Its guiding principles are based on current science and relevant research is available, *inter alia*, with the following aspects relevant to patient safety:

The Constitution of the World Health Organization states

- The enjoyment of the highest attainable standard of health is one of the fundamental rights of every human being without distinction of race, religion, political belief, economic or social condition.

- The health of all peoples is fundamental to the attainment of peace and security and is dependent upon the fullest co-operation of individuals and States.
- The achievement of any State in the promotion and protection of health is of value to all.
- Unequal development in different countries in the promotion of health and control of disease, especially communicable disease, is a common danger (WHO, 2020).

(https://www.who.int/about/governance/constitution)

Patient-centred decision-making and safety

The normal expectation of service users is a positive experience, which is based on safe standards of care during their patient journey. At the centre of any decision-making should be the patient with the aim to keep them safe. They (patients) do not anticipate being victims of harm due to clinicians' negligent actions, omissions or recklessness. High expectations may at times be dashed when things may go wrong. Due to human factors, one can never guarantee eliminating risk, only minimise it to an acceptable level. The Hippocratic Oath still has relevance in current healthcare practice, Bioethics and patient safety as summarised in the principles below.

- Of solidarity with teachers and other physicians.
- Of beneficence (to do good or avoid evil) and non-maleficence (from the Latin 'primum non nocere', or 'do no harm') towards patients. (In fact, the well-known 'first do no harm' phrase does not feature in the classical Hippocratic Oath.)
- Not to assist suicide or abortion.
- To leave surgery to surgeons.
- Not to harm, especially not to seduce patients.
- To maintain confidentiality and never to gossip.

(Hurwitz and Richardson, 1997)

Regrettably, there have been occasions when things have gone wrong when patients have been harmed by the actions of healthcare professionals and/or due to systems failures or shortcomings in practice related to the conduct of healthcare staff.

Based on evolving medical science, one example of evolving practice is cardiopulmonary resuscitation (CPR). Over time, CPR underwent a variety of what can only be considered today as unorthodox and unsafe practice CPR. During the Middle Ages, one example was the use of bellows by Parcelsus, the Swiss physician ((1530). Subsequently, the standard practice developed in time on the back of what may be seen as, 'unsafe, ineffective, or outright dangerous' today. The CPR procedure as it evolved and was considered safe then, with the following timeline.

Timeline of the development of cardiopulmonary resuscitation

1700s: 1740 – Mouth-to-mouth resuscitation was officially recommended for drowning victims by The French Academy of Sciences (French: Académie des Sciences) in Paris.

1767 – The Society for the Recovery of Drowned Persons became the first organised effort to deal with sudden and unexpected death.

1800s: 1891 – Dr. Friedrich Maass performed the first equivocally documented chest compression in humans.

1900s: 1903 – Dr. George Crile reported the first successful use of external chest compressions in human resuscitation.

1904 – Dr. George Crile performed the first American case of closed-chest cardiac massage.

1954 – James Elam was the first to prove that expired air was sufficient to maintain adequate oxygenation; CPR invented (USA).

1956 – Peter Safar and James Elam invented mouth-to-mouth resuscitation.

(ProCPR; https://www.procpr.org/blog/misc/history-of-cpr)

Even with advanced technology, the risk though minimised will still exist. It is a question of how low it is permissible, and that is the challenge for clinicians. Despite the best intention, it is possible that there may be system failures or human factors. Things may go wrong, and patients may be harmed needlessly.

Unfortunately, there have also been several cases when healthcare staff were negligent or committed crimes and were in breach of the trust bestowed upon them by becoming perpetrators themselves and deliberately harming patients. Other healthcare personnel may be privy to harmful situations and in fact choose to be indifferent bystanders, doing nothing to stop avoidable harm to vulnerable service users or advocate for them. A recent example is the Lucy Letby case, where a paediatric nurse was convicted on seven counts of murder and counts of manslaughter of at least six neonatal babies. Questions may be asked as to how much her colleagues knew and why they did nothing.

Harm is inevitably linked to human factors either directly or indirectly. This includes deviation from standards or norm, due to negligence or recklessness, incompetent staff or wilful criminal actions. There may be consequences, with near misses or resulting harm to patients. Healthcare professionals and other care staff are accountable for their actions.

It is not possible to guarantee a 100% safe outcome due to human factors. The objective for the healthcare professional should be risk assessment and management, thus minimising risk. Several risk assessment tools are available in clinical practice for various specialities. It is also important for healthcare providers to monitor near misses or never events which in fact are avoidable. Clinicians should aim to reduce risk manage, with review dates for checking the effectiveness of a given plan to see if it is working or if a change of interventions is required. A care plan review or evaluation should provide an opportunity for keeping any planned interventions in place if they are working, discontinue the interventions and amend if the goal has been met. If it turns out to be the case that it is not working, then there may be a case for changing to a different intervention. The question arises as to whether any level of interventions can ever be deemed as a guarantee for safety, given that human factors are always present.

Patient-centred decision-making, rights for vulnerable people

The same principles of safety may be applicable to all specialist areas of practice.

The above landmark case introduced the 'neighbour principle' in Donoghue v Stevenson (1932).

UKHL 100, a Scottish case which was decided in the House of Lords to become the cornerstone of the 'marriage' between law and ethics.

Case Law: Donoghue v Stevenson (1932) UKHL 100

On 26 August 1928, Mrs Donoghue's friend bought her a ginger-beer from Wellmeadow Café in Paisley. She consumed about half of the bottle, which was made of dark opaque glass, when the remainder of the contents was poured into a tumbler. At this point, the decomposed remains of a snail floated out, causing her alleged shock and severe gastro-enteritis.

Mrs Donoghue was not able to claim through breach of warranty of a contract: she was not party to any contract. Therefore, she issued proceedings against Stevenson, the manufacture, which snaked its way up to the House of Lords.

(https://www.lawteacher.net/cases/donoghue-v-stevenson.php)

Lord Atkins applied ethical principles to develop the Common law duty of care (to be explored in Chapter 3). The ethical and legal framework requires clinicians to ensure that service.

Users in their care are not harmed by their negligent actions or omissions. This case also established the so-called 'Neighbour Principle' which underpins the 'duty of care' concept now applicable to Tort Law (which includes clinical negligence claims).

The 'neighbour principle' is defined by Lord Atkins:

Who, then, in law, is my neighbour? The answer seems to be—persons who are so closely and directly affected by my act that I ought reasonably to have them in contemplation as being so affected when I am directing my mind to the acts or omissions which are called in question.

(Lord Atkins, *Donoghue* v Stevenson (1932), UKHL 100)

Based on the above-mentioned principle of law, it is easy to see any meaningful partnership in decision-making. The Bioethical principle of 'To do no harm', the standard of accountability for clinicians' negligent actions or omissions, has been adopted by healthcare professional codes of conduct.

The Common Law of Tort, and Scots Law of Delict, a duty of care (in Donoghue case, above) is now enshrined in the Health and Safety at Work Act (HASAWA, 1974. The responsibilities of any employer who owns or has responsible for any premises or settings are clearly defined as a duty of care in Health and Safety law (please see Chapter 2). As it stands, Articles of the European Convention on Human Rights (1950) enshrines any person's rights are not infringed by others' actions. A healthcare provider has a duty of care to ensure the safety of all who enter their premises, under sections 2 and 3 of HASAWA (1974). An employee on the other hand also has a duty of care to ensure the safety and wellbeing of all who enter any given healthcare providing premises, as clearly defined in section 7 of HASAWA (1974). This will also be applied in subsequent chapters. The main themes to be explored will therefore be applicable to clinicians from all disciplines of healthcare. Health and safety law applies to all work-related environments including institutions or the community.

Some groups of service users are more vulnerable than others. Healthcare professionals have a moral and legal obligation to ensure that they safeguard service users and advocate for their rights. This is necessary for the safety of service users or patients, especially those who are at a higher risk. Healthcare professionals are required to improve their own knowledge and awareness of health and safety and the impact of human factors.

It is essential that healthcare professionals acquire proficiency in producing evidence that can be used for making improvements to patient's safety and managing the risks of adverse events.

(Donaldson et al., 2020, p. 3)

Clinicians and healthcare staff owe a duty of care to ensure that all patients or colleagues are not harmed by their negligent actions or omissions. Whistleblowing and safeguarding are key tools for advocacy and for protecting vulnerable groups. Advocacy is important and an opportunity for healthcare professionals to champion the human rights and safeguard vulnerable people. This applies to marginalised groups and/or those who fall under the umbrella of those with 'protected characteristics' subject to section 4 of the Equality Act (2010), Buka (2020). Equality legislation was in response to meeting the need for protection of vulnerable people who may also be marginalised. The lynchpin for promoting a culture of safety must be based on inclusion in healthcare provision (please confer in Chapter 3). Consequently, this means that individuals who fall within the classification of protected characteristics may be victims of discrimination and hence their level of risk could therefore be higher than that of those who may not be subject to discrimination.

One example of key areas of practice has been that of drafting clinical guidelines for safety in operating theatres, thus minimising errors, near misses and adverse events. The WHO has a wider remit in stipulating guidelines on safe management of certain conditions. For example, this has been clearly the case when related to guidelines for managing pandemics such as those for COVID. The advice they followed had been reportedly science-driven. National governments may, in turn, adopt these guidelines at their own national levels.

The HASAWA (1974) remains the pivotal piecemeal legislation developed for safety in any work-related and other environments where people may engage. This statute and its subordinate regulations became key to health and safety as applicable to different settings in the United Kingdom. In 1974, John Locke became the first Director General for the Health and Safety Executive. Statutory provisions will be applied in subsequent chapters.

In due course, the term Clinical Governance was introduced by the Department of Health White Paper, The New NHS: Modern, Dependable (1998) (to be explored in Chapter 2). This was aimed at improving the quality and setting standards of care as well as highlighting the need to improve patient safety. A relatively recent development was in 2021 when a National Patient Safety Committee was set up, with the remit to provide:

> a strategic role in considering the existing landscape of national patient safety planning, response and improvement and consistently share insight and thinking about how, as a national healthcare system, we can improve the effectiveness of these patient safety functions.
>
> (https://www.england.nhs.uk/patient-safety/
> the-national-patient-safety-committee/)

Patients are more likely to be vulnerable due to their condition and dependence. Vulnerability may be related to their physical and mental health. As acknowledged above, the patient–clinician relationship is fiduciary (i.e., based on trust) and, therefore, an unequal one. This can be seen as one of power or control on the part of the clinician versus dependence for the patient. Though well-meaning, such a relationship is clearly unbalanced and may reinforce the Paternalism theory. Regardless of how well meant this may be, it would be potentially disempowering for the patient or service user. The NHS Constitution (2012), as updated in 2021, however, goes to the heart of promoting patient-choice and shared decision-making as well as the patient's human right to choose which is based on:

Right to respect for private and family life

1 Everyone has the right to respect for his private and family life, his home and his correspondence.

> (Article 8, European Convention on Human Rights (1950))

The challenge, however, remains for all clinicians working with service users in a variety of settings. The latter may lack capacity for decision-making as defined by the Mental Capacity Act 2005. There are nevertheless exceptions under the Mental Health Act (1983), subject to which compulsory admissions may be allowed. Those who lack mental capacity may have their freedom deprived in their 'best interests'. subject to DoLS, to be replaced by Liberty Protection Safeguards.

Treatment therapies and medicines management and administration to patients should have positive outcomes with benefits; nevertheless, there may also be and always a risk, hence a need for appropriate monitoring. It is therefore important for clinicians to follow procedures for safeguarding vulnerable patients. The most reliable way is being guided by national or local guidelines using the relevant assessment tools on all aspects of care. To identify patients who may be at a higher risk so something can be done about it. Examples could be work practices resourcing and staff training, which could impact vulnerable patients at risk. It is also important for the employer to secure satisfactory and regular background checks for Disclosure and Barring Service (DBS) on backgrounds of staff caring for vulnerable patients, as well as safe and secure medicines and medicinal products access, storage and dispensing. The needs of vulnerable people such as children and frail and elderly patients or those with mental health needs require even closer monitoring.

One example of significant note is systems failure in the case of Dr Shipman (1971–2001), a former (sole practice) GP who was responsible for the deaths of over 250 vulnerable people, mainly elderly, though there were a few younger victims who were harmed by his actions. This case highlighted a systems failure and poor communication between agencies including healthcare staff such as pharmacists, community nurses, social workers and funeral directors. The recommendations of the enquiries aimed at minimising this and at shared decision-making with patients.

Thinking Point

1 Identify one example of risk assessment and risk management tool that you undertake in your workplace.
2 List 2 aspects in which you would like to see some improvement in?
3 If you were an employer of healthcare staff, what additional measure would you recommend ensuring that you improve the safety of patients in your care – list 2–3?

Conclusion

This chapter introduces the concept of patient safety. There was consideration of background issues on a broad topic applicable to patient safety, within any given healthcare context. The background to safety is complex. Due to the nature of this broad topic, there are many different facets which may be applicable to many settings related to health and social care provisions (which may be overlapping depending on the service user's needs).

Hopefully, this chapter will also have served as an introduction and groundwork setting challenges while motivating readers who are healthcare clinicians and learners. It is hoped that the reader will explore and reflect on key issues while exploring the challenges posed by health and safety considerations. This is especially pertinent in respect of assessing and managing risk for a diverse population of vulnerable service users. Thereafter, the reader is encouraged to focus on aspects of safety as it affects patients while exploring the ethico-legal implications of inadequate risk assessments and any breaches of key safety statutory and professional regulatory requirements.

References

Beauchamp TL, Childress JF (2019) *Principles of biomedical ethics* (8th ed.). Oxford, Oxford University Press

Buka P (2020) *Essential law and ethics, patients, rights, and decision-making in nursing* (3rd ed.). Abington, Routledge

County Asylums Act (1808)

Donaldson L, Ricciardi W, Sheridan S, Tartaglia R, eds. (2020) *Textbook of patient safety and clinical risk management.* Cham, Springer Open Access

Donoghue v Stevenson (1932) UKHL 100

Equality Act (2010)

Employers Liability Act (1969)

European Convention on Human Rights (1950). The Convention in 1950. Available online at: https://www.coe.int/en/web/human-rights-convention/the-convention-in-1950

Factory Act (1833)

Factory Act (1844)

Geezer Retro (2021) Your life in their hands, Geezer, Retro. "Your Life in Their Hands | Nostalgia Central" (Accessed on 6th January 2021)

GMC (2019) Good medical practice; General medical council

Health and Safety at Work Act (1974) sections 2, 3 and 7. Health and Safety at Work etc Act 1974. Available online at: https://www.hse.gov.uk/legislation/hswa.htm

Human Rights Act (1998) Available online at: https://www.legislation.gov.uk/ukpga/1998/42/contents

Hurd D (2007) *Robert Peel: A biography.* London, Orion Publishing.

Hurwitz B, Richardson R (1997) Swearing to care: The resurgence in medical oaths. BMJ.

Mental Health Act (1959) Available online at: https://www.legislation.gov.uk/ukpga/Eliz2/7-8/72

Mental Health Act (1983) Available online at: https://www.legislation.gov.uk/ukpga/1983/20/contents

Mental Health (2007) Available online at: https://www.legislation.gov.uk/ukpga/2007/12/contents

NHS Patient Safety Strategy (2021) DoH. Available online at: https://www.england.nhs.uk/patient-safety/the-nhs-patient-safety-strategy/ (Accessed on 22nd October 2023)

NHS Constitution (2012, 2019) NHS Constitution for England. Available online at: https://www.gov.uk/government/publications/the-nhs-constitution-for-england

Priestley v Fowler [1837] 150 ER 1030

Sanai L (2006 Jan 7) A history of Britain's hospitals and the background to the medical, nursing and allied professions. BMJ, 332(7532), 57

WHO (2020) Constitution of the World Health Organization, article 2, j-t. Available online at: https://apps.who.int/gb/bd/pdf_files/BD_49th-en.pdf (Accessed on 20th October 2023)

WHO (2023) Patient safety. Available online at: https://www.who.int/news-room/fact-sheets/detail/patient-safety

2 Clinical governance, risk and human factors

Paul Buka and Cheyne Truman

Introduction

The early 1990s witnessed development of policy which was more focused on patient safety, with introduction of the concept of 'clinical governance' or quality of care'. This should be a vehicle for delivery of care 'safely'. The Labour government introduced this in 1992 with a focus on improving patient safety aimed at reducing harm to patients. Risk management, one of the pillars of clinical governance, is key to keeping patients safe.

Patient safety is defined as "the absence of preventable harm to a patient and reduction of risk of unnecessary harm associated with health care to an acceptable minimum" (WHO, 2023).

Clinical governance, quality of care, risk and patient safety

Quality in the National Health Service (NHS) was later defined in three elements as set out below by Lord Darzi Report (2008). Clinical governance has since been the basis of quality of care, with the three cornerstones in the NHS. These should follow the three elements, as identified below.

1 Safe
2 Effective, with
3 Positive patient experience.

> (Department of Health, 2008, p. 47;
> http://www.dh.gov.uk/prod_consum_dh/groups/dh_digitalassets/
> @dh/@en/documents/digitalasset/dh_085828.pdf)

The government introduced the term 'clinical governance' with seven 'pillars' for signposting key aspects of quality at improvement of care (The Health of the Nation, 1992) as a framework for accountability. Other factors contributing to the rise in litigation by victims of clinical negligence may be the fact that people are more informed these days. The Citizen's Charter (1991) also aimed to make healthcare providers more accountable.

DOI: 10.4324/9781003376934-2

Since the launch of clinical governance, there has been an increased awareness of patient safety, with more accountability. This means that healthcare providers now need to be better prepared, with a drive towards restructuring the NHS systems and processes (so they are fit for purpose) with a positive outcome related to patient safety. With demographic changes and an increase in life expectancy, there will be more people requiring healthcare with potentially more with co-morbidities.

Clinical governance means that potential victims of clinical negligence are becoming more aware of their rights. We are now living in a litigious society, with civil actions for personal injury more likely. There is therefore now a need for an improved focus on healthcare and health promotion and patients' safety.

A significant move in improving patient safety was the setting up of the National Patient Safety Agency in 2001. This was responsible for establishing a 'national reporting and learning system for adverse events' (NPSA, 2001). The aim was to learn from the reports as well as develop solutions to prevent, and reduce, the risk of such events happening again. One example was the need for training in safe equipment usage for staff. In the face of such challenges, service users became more aware of their rights and therefore likely to complain formally and/or litigate for personal injury resulting from clinical negligence. Like most western societies with an advanced economy, the United Kingdom has become an increasingly litigious society, with many claims being settled out of court.

Healthcare providers should aim to deliver patient-centred care to minimise risk. This means that treatment and decision-making should afford the patient a sufficient degree of information to enable them to decide. This is described as:

> ... a process whereby a patient is supported to articulate what they hope treatment or support to self-manage will achieve; the patient is informed about the benefits and risks of any treatment or support options available; the patient and clinician arrive at a decision based on mutual understanding and the decision made is recorded and then implemented.
>
> (Coulter and Collins, 2011)

Litigation against the NHS had been on the increase, doubling between 1990 and 1998, during which time hospital activity had increased by 30%. The overall expenditure on clinical negligence by the NHS in 1998 was then estimated to be more than £84 million (Fenn et al., 2000).

More recent figures from the NHS Resolution (2022/23) show that litigation for personal injury in the NHS has been on the rise, with the total cost for all clinical schemes for 2020/21 as high as £2,209.3 million (£2,402 million in 2021/22) in total. Legal costs and lawyers' fees for both sides can be substantial and as high as 40% of the total costs (NHS Resolution, 2022/23) (see Chapter 4). The 6Cs (Care, Compassion, Competence, Communication, Courage and Commitment), all values essential to high-quality care (NHS Professionals, no date), have now been updated and since superseded by the 7Ps. They include public and patient safety (Nursing Times 16 November 2023 ed.), which also focuses on 'patient-centred care'.

Since October 2023, the Health Services Safety Investigations Body (HSSIB) is an independent arm's length body of the Department of Health and Social Care, under Health and Social Care Act (2022), which aimed to develop integrated care.

It investigates patient safety concerns nationally in both the NHS (England) and in independent healthcare settings with a focus on safety learning and improving quality of care.

Our investigations aim to reduce patient harm by:

- Supporting the involvement of patients, families and carers in healthcare.
- Supporting healthcare staff to carry out their roles and care for patients safely.
- Creating safer healthcare environments and processes.
- Making healthcare services more efficient.
- Sharing best practice and innovations in patient care.

(Healthcare Safety Investigation Branch, 2023; https://www.hssib.org.uk/)

The UK countries still have the Healthcare Safety Investigation Branch (HSIB) in place.

Human factors, risk assessment and root cause analysis

The Health and Safety at Work Act (HASAWA, 1974), sections 2 and 7 place a duty of care (on the employer and employee respectively) to ensure the safety of persons, including patients and staff or visitors, in any given clinical setting. Furthermore, the Management of Health and Safety at Work Regulations 1999, regulation 5 requires 'employers to plan, organise and control monitoring and review'. This includes measures for risk assessment and management.

A risk assessment should be followed by control measures with the aim of not eliminating but minimising and managing any given risk.

- Identify hazards.
- Assess the risks.
- Control the risks.
- Record your findings.
- Review the controls.

(HSE, managing risks and risk assessment at work; https://www.hse.gov.uk/simple-health-safety/risk/ steps-needed-to-manage-risk.htm)

The term 'Human Factors', also called 'Ergonomics', is a discipline which echoes the physical and psychological aspects of individuals as well as organisations in relation to safety and risk assessment. This is also "… environmental, organisational and job factors, and human and individual characteristics, which influence behaviour at work in a way which can affect health and safety" (Royal College of Radiologists, 2019). People or occupiers injured on healthcare premises may also be covered by occupiers' liability under the Occupier's Liability Acts 1957 and 1984, which cover visitors and trespassers respectively in England and Wales, or by the Occupier's Liability (Scotland) Act 1960.

This area is linked to structural factors which are imbedded within procedures of a given organisational system or environment. It is important for healthcare providers to learn from events. Reason (1990) pioneered the explanation of the occurrence of systems breakdown, which are due to resource failures and human errors.

HSE guidance of any given activity or task considers three key elements:

* the job or task in hand,
* the individual or person responsible, as well as
* the organisation in which this takes place (HSE, 1991).

Teamwork is therefore crucial, and team members should be aware of their roles and what is going on. *Inter alia*, poor communication could be an issue resulting in patients being harmed. (Please see the following case and also Chapter 8 on team roles). This is also subject to The Workplace (Health Safety and Welfare) Regulations 1992.

Case Study: The Bromiley Case: Parliamentary Select Committee on Health Report (2008)

Elaine Bromiley went into hospital for a routine sinus operation and during anaesthetic induction, it all went horribly wrong. Her airway obstructed and the team was unable to gain a secure airway. For 20 minutes they attempted to achieve a stable airway, during which time her oxygen saturations were around 40%. Although she survived, she sustained serious hypoxic brain injury and 13 days later her life support was turned off. Martin (her husband) was an airline pilot with an interest in human factors and he subsequently formed the Clinical Human Factors Group in 2007.

One of the main teamwork lessons from Elaine's case was communication.

Communication between team members is crucial, and in Elaine's case, the communication process dried up completely. There were three senior and experienced doctors in the room – two anaesthetic consultants and an ENT consultant. They did not communicate with each other, and nobody vocalised what was happening (i.e. this patient is in trouble, this is a 'can't intubate, can't ventilate' situation).

(Select Committee on Health Written Evidence, Memorandum by the Clinical Human Factors Group (CHFG) (PS 24), https://publications.parliament.uk/pa/cm200708/cmselect/cmhealth/1137/1137we25.htm)

Risk assessment is necessary in order to identify hazards and to determine the likelihood of a specific undesirable event occurring. This is achieved through risk control measures Regulation 5, which applies to maintenance of equipment in efficient working order. This should help in prevention of future adverse events.

Thinking Point (in respect of the Bromley case)

1 Identify the main communication issues in the above case.
2 What recommendations would you make in order to minimise the likelihood of such a catastrophic failure happening again?

Major injury or ill health which occurs in any given work environment must be reported to the HSE, subject to the Reporting of Injuries, Diseases and Dangerous Occurrences Regulations (RIDDOR, 2013). In the aftermath of any such adverse event, an internal investigation normally led by a line manager and a workplace health and safety representative is required by law.

A root cause analysis should take place after the event, and it is important, as a learning point, to establish what happened. Serious events, including acts, omissions, unexpected or avoidable injury or death, and near misses and never events which prevent or threaten an organisation's delivery, must also be investigated. These may be clinical or non-clinical and obviously the latter may indirectly impact patients. An example is data breaches, or staff member injury due to trips and falls, resulting in injury and absence from work. This may have direct or indirect effect on the quality of healthcare delivery. Any subsequent investigation should focus on cause and effect.

The NHS Serious Incident Framework (2015) has been superseded by a new system which aims at a more patient-centred approach, the Patient Safety Incident Response Framework (PSIRF, 2022). Its focus is on engagement and involvement of patients, families and staff, following a patient safety incident. This should be based on the following engagement principles:

1 Apologies are meaningful.
2 Approach is individualised.
3 Timing is sensitive.
4 Those affected are treated with respect.
5 Guidance and clarity are provided.
6 Those affected are heard.
7 Approach is collaborative.
8 Subjectivity is accepted.
9 Strive for equity.

(Patient Safety Incident Response Framework supporting guidance, 2022, https://www.england.nhs.uk/patient-safety/patient-safety-insight/incident-response-framework/)

This applies to service providers.

The Medicines and Healthcare Regulatory Authority (MHRA) – updated the Central Alerting System (CAS) patient safety warnings in 2022. This is a 'a web-based cascading system' for issuing patient safety alerts, 'important public health messages and other safety critical information and guidance to the NHS'. Independent providers of health and social care providers also have access (MHRA, 2024).

Risk assessment is necessary, not only to identify hazards but to eliminate them where possible. The next stage would be to minimise risk to an acceptable level. Human factors as identified by Reason (1990) in the Swiss Cheese Model, any which identifies elements which may cause as:

1 Organisational influences,
2 Unsafe supervision,
3 Preconditions for unsafe acts, and
4 The unsafe acts themselves.

(James Reason Swiss Cheese Model,
https://skybrary.aero/articles/james-reason-hf-model)

The Swiss Cheese Model theory Reason (1990) follows a systems approach and is broadly applicable to any sector where people work, such as factories, offices, building sites, transport like the aviation industry as well as hospitals and healthcare provision environments. Medical or surgical mishaps also fall into this category, where human errors may affect the outcome. For example, following any investigation when things went wrong, a recommendation on how best to reduce harm to patients for the future would be appropriate.

Human factors may allow room for error. Based on Reason's Swiss Cheese Model, however, where failings or loopholes appear within an organisation, patients may be harmed. There is nevertheless always room for improvement and for lessons to be learnt from adverse events.

The Swiss Cheese model as applied to healthcare, stated simply, postulates that errors and means for the prevention of errors are multifactorial, and that a number of possibilities for error will usually be offset by a number of layers of defences'.

(CCF0010 – Evidence on NHS Complaints and Clinical Failure,
https://committees.parliament.uk/writtenevidence/55955/
html/#:~:text=The%20Swiss%20Cheese%20model%
20as,number%20of%20layers%20of%20defences)

An alternative assessment tool for root cause analysis of human factors is one identified by the Royal College of Nursing (RCN) Wheel. This focuses on human factors and how actions or omissions may result in performance or lapses may adversely affect a patient. In this model the patient sits, literally at the centre of the wheel. This represents a patient-centred approach to safe health delivery with a focus on safe systems of work. The updated RCN Wheel (2019) is associated with the Leadership Management and Quality (LMQ) Human Factors Model (1993), which was developed for teams. Airline pilots were the focus, though other teams such as healthcare and railway management use this model in order to improve patient or customer safety. For example, one context was improving training to enhance performance and to develop standards and programmes for flight crews, traffic controllers and engineers.

If things go wrong, the NHS may follow a root cause analysis (as discussed below) as a structured method of analysing serious adverse events. The aim should not be to identify culprits, apportion blame or punish the alleged 'wrongdoer', but rather to learn from the events while putting in place preventative procedures so the error does not happen again. It should be more about learning lessons, so the event does not happen again.

Another alternative in use is the Cause-and-Effect Fishbone or Ishikawa (1968) diagram, which was first developed in Japan. This follows process mapping, taking into account essential elements such as the Environment, Methods, Equipment and People, linking this to the problem or outcome.

There are three basic types of root causes that can have a potential impact on a problem, such as:

- Physical causes: May arise due to problems with any physical component of a system, such as hardware failure and equipment malfunction.
- Human causes: May occur due to human error, caused by lack of skills and knowledge to perform a task.
- Organisational causes: May happen when organisations use a system or process that is faulty or insufficient, in situations like giving incomplete instructions, making wrong decisions and mishandling staff and property.

(Safety Culture, 2023,
https://safetyculture.com/topics/root-cause-analysis/)

When things go wrong, patient advocacy and whistle blowing

In the aftermath of the Mid-Staffordshire Trust scandal, the subsequent Mid Staffordshire NHS Foundation Trust Public Inquiry (2013), identified organisational failures and raised the level of public awareness of the need for safety and safeguarding vulnerable patients. In June 2014, a government campaign was launched with an aim to improve standards with "… a three-year shared objective to save 6,000 lives and halve avoidable harm as part of our journey towards ensuring patients get harm free care every time, everywhere" (Sign up to Safety, 2014, updated in 2018). This was also in response to the Berwick Report (2013), which had highlighted patient safety issues while aiming to reduce harm to patients and therefore save lives.

Some progress has been made in the development of policies related to raising clinical governance awareness; nevertheless, this remains a challenge in all care sectors, with a few cases of abuse of vulnerable patients especially persons who lack capacity or have mental health needs. The Winterbourne View case is in point.

Case Study: Winterbourne View 2011

Forty safeguarding alerts were made concerning Winterbourne View patients from October 2007-April 2011: 27 allegations of staff-to-patient assaults and, ten allegations of patient-to-patient assaults and three family-related alerts. But in only 19 cases were service users who were the subject of alerts seen by the police or social workers with the other 21 largely left to Castlebeck to investigate. "Unprofessional behaviour" by staff, written complaints by patients, escalating self-harm … including 379 incidences recorded in 2010 and 129 in the first three months of 2011.

The review found that social workers and other safeguarding staff treated these as discrete incidents and failed to identify a pattern of concern at the hospital; they also relied too much on Winterbourne's management to honestly report the facts concerning referrals.

(https://www.communitycare.co.uk/2012/08/07/winterbourne-view-a-case-study-in-institutional-abuse/)

Thinking Point

Service user A speaks to you in confidence and makes allegations of psychological abuse by B who is a staff member. They, however, do not wish to let anyone else know, for fear of repercussion,

1 How do you deal with this matter?
2 If the person in question happens to be your line manager, how would you manage this situation?
3 What is the whistleblowing policy in your employing organisation?

Sir Robert Francis' Freedom to Speak Up Review (2015) followed the Francis Report (2013).

This was in the aftermath of the Mid-Staffordshire Report. In an ideal world, staff should feel free to speak about concerns on patient safety. Sir Robert Francis set out up to 20 principles, aiming to generate conditions, including those conducive to speaking up and, *inter alia*, support for openness and for staff to speak up without fear of consequences. Cultural organisations with issues such as bullying and toxicity and fear of managers may result in staff doing nothing due to a 'bystanders' effect' response.

Following any given event, staff may be fearful of exposing or speaking out in case this jeopardises their career.

Case Study: Wrong Operation Site

A patient underwent surgery on the wrong wrist: A Foundation Year 2 doctor noted that she thought the consultant surgeon was preparing the wrong hand for surgery, however, all staff were progressing as if this was the correct wrist. The Foundation Year 2 doctor made an attempt to raise the concern with the registrar, but this was not registered, and the Foundation Year 2 doctor was asked quite bluntly to remain quiet. The surgical incision was made, and the operation started. After ten minutes it was noted that the injury for which the child was undergoing the operation was not present. The operation was then undertaken on the correct side. The child suffered some pain, discomfort and scarring on the wrongly operated side, but made a good recovery.

What happened? The Foundation Year 2 doctor was very fearful of raising a concern due to the hierarchical nature of the organisation and as she had been reprimanded before for a failure to get a patient investigated promptly. The Foundation Year 2 doctor was unsure how to raise concerns and challenge authority and felt a significant amount of guilt about her inability to raise this concern.

(Human Factors in Healthcare A Concordat from the National Quality Board, https://www.england.nhs.uk/wp-content/uploads/2013/11/nqb-hum-fact-concord.pdf)

It is possible to remove a hazard; however, regarding an identifiable risk, it is only a question of minimising it and the likelihood of its recurrence. It should be possible to learn from experience through root cause analysis. By asking the '5 Whys' to hopefully find some answers to the cause of an adverse event. The '5 Whys' is a simple tool commonly used to assess the root cause analysis in the NHS. It starts by aiming to explore a statement (e.g., why did the surgeon operate on the wrong limb?). This should help investigators understand and establish the outcome. This can be used during or after an event in the NHS. The '5 Whys' model was developed in the car manufacturing industry in the 1970s (Birt, 2023).

The following case demonstrated the fact that proactive interventions can work and that doing nothing is not an option.

Case Study: 13 Patient Safety First: Reducing Harm From Deterioration Intervention – NHS Somerset 27 Project: To Reduce the Number of Falls in Community Hospitals

Rationale...

In 2007, the National Patient Safety Association reported that 28,000 falls were reported in community hospitals each year. This was a pertinent issue for NHS Somerset within newly built hospitals where patients had their own bathrooms, making them less visible to nursing staff. Approach: An audit was performed in one of the pilot hospitals to find out exactly when and where falls were taking place. It was found that the majority were happening during the night, so regular 15-minute walk rounds for the nursing staff were initiated so that they could check if patients were wandering out of their beds and looked unstable - or if they had fallen and had not already been helped.

The PDSA (Plan-Do-Study-Act) cycles, as recommended by Patient Safety First, was used to test out the changes.

(Human Factors in Healthcare, A Concordant from the National Quality Board, https://www.england.nhs.uk/wp-content/uploads/2013/11/nqb-hum-fact-concord.pdf)

Patient advocacy is a prerequisite for the fiduciary relationship between patient and clinician. All professional codes of conduct highlight the need for clinicians to be aware of patient's vulnerability. However, there is now a requirement for a duty of candour (Francis Report, 2013) for staff to be open in practice. All staff should feel free to raise any concerns with managers or organisational speak-up guardians. It can be difficult for an internal investigation to be conducted anonymously. Alternatively, staff may raise any concerns externally, with the CQC or HSE without compromising anonymity. In practice, it can be intimidating for staff to raise any concerns. The impact on staff welfare and wellbeing cannot be underestimated (see Chapter 7).

Thinking Point

Professional Codes of conduct for healthcare clinicians require advocacy vulnerable patients and speaking out for those less able to assert their own rights.

• How far would you go to ensure advocacy for those vulnerable patients especially those less able to speak for themselves?

The 'Bystander effect' theory refers to 'the inhibiting influence of the presence of others on a person's willingness to help someone in need' (Britannica, 2024). This could suggest compromising advocacy for vulnerable patients. This means that staff who happen to witness or be privy to patient safety issues may hide behind a toxic or negative culture within a team or organisation and therefore do nothing. This may be due to fear of repercussion, victimisation or being targeted by the person or persons associated including managers within a healthcare organisation (see Chapter 8).

> Scores of experiments have shown that people are much less likely to intervene in an emergency, and are generally slower to respond, when other people are present than when they are alone, and this phenomenon is sometimes called group inhibition of helping. It was discovered by US psychologists Bibb Latané (born 1937) and John Mc Connon Darley (born 1938).
> (Oxford Reference, https://www.oxfordreference.com/
> display/10.1093/oi/authority.20110803095539861)

It is possible that some staff may feel intimidated and not be comfortable or courageous enough to raise concerns due to fear of retribution, as highlighted above. Nevertheless, due to duty of care, there could also be potential negligence and/or professional misconduct implications for failing to advocate for vulnerable patients.

> A 2013 NHS staff survey showed that only 72% of respondents were confident that it is safe to raise a concern. There are disturbing reports of what happens to those who do raise concerns. Yet failure to speak up can cost lives.
> (Francis, 2015, para. 1, p. 3, http://freedomtospeakup.
> org.uk/wp-content/uploads/2014/07/F2SU_web.pdf)

There have also been documented cases of toxic cultures like bullying, this may generate fear and poor staff morale. The Mid-Staffordshire Case (2013) discussed above is an example and, more recently, the Lucy Letby Case (2022). There have been cases where whistle-blowers faced real consequences of victimisation and threats to their employment status (see Chapter 7).

Case Study: Police Investigating Dozens of Patient Deaths at Hospital in Brighton

Police are investigating dozens of deaths at the Royal Sussex County Hospital in Brighton over a five-year period, after two senior consultant surgeons who raised patient safety concerns were dismissed from their jobs.

Krishna Singh and Mansoor Foroughi are bringing employment tribunal claims against University Hospitals Sussex NHS Foundation Trust, which runs the hospital, after losing their jobs. Singh, a general surgeon, was clinical director for abdominal surgery and medicine, and Foroughi, a neurosurgeon, specialises in brain and spine surgery.

The *Guardian*, which broke the story, reported that the number of deaths is around 40. A statement from Sussex Police said that the force had "received allegations of medical negligence at the Royal Sussex County Hospital, Brighton, and is currently assessing these allegations".

(Dyer, 2023)

To improve communication and collaboration of healthcare providers, the new Health and Care Act (2022), 'removes barriers which stop the system from being truly integrated, with different parts of the NHS working better together, alongside local government, to tackle the nation's health inequalities. Secondly, the Act reduces bureaucracy across the system'.

Moving and handling safely

Moving and handling people in healthcare is carried out day to day, but if not done safely can result in serious injury. Numerous moving and handling legislation (listed below) are designed to protect those involved, and to minimise risk to all, including, patients, staff and members of the public.

- Health and Safety at Work Act 1974 (HASAWA)
- Manual Handling Operations Regulations 1992 (MHOR) (as amended 2002)
- The Management of Health and Safety at Work Regulations 1999
- Provision and Use of Work Equipment Regulations 1998 (PUWER)
- Lifting Operations and Lifting Regulations 1998 (LOLER)

Duties are set out according to employer and employee contracts and terms of employment. The above regulations embrace duty of care with training, compliance, reporting and recording protocols. The core aim is embedded in safety, risk minimising and harm avoidance as well as occupational health. There is a need for regulation. Risk assessment is a key part of regulation, with provision and maintenance of appropriate equipment. It is not enough for an employer or workplace to provide equipment to mitigate risk and improve work safety without regular risk-assessing, servicing and maintenance of said equipment. Equally, provision of this equipment is irrelevant without proper training and use thereof.

NHS Resolution (2020) cites 4,733 manual handling-related claims of which 2,008 were settled with around £57.1m paid out in damages and legal costs over a ten-year period. At least 45% of those settled relate to back injuries. Ultimately, despite the varying reasons, the consensus refers to 'inadequate training, risk assessments and equipment'. Also noted as causes are inadequate application of training, risk assessments and equipment. Overall, the report revealed many incidents involving the movement of people but also use of clinical and non-clinical equipment.

Familiarity with equipment manuals or attending training alone is insufficient. Staff have a duty of care to ensure application. The NMC (2018) requires nurses to work only within their competence and not carry out tasks they are not trained to do. The same also applies under the regulations listed above. As technology advances, equipment changes; therefore, when moving from one workplace to another the operators of equipment must be trained in what they are to do. However aside from the equipment alone, patients are individuals, and each comes with their own knowledge, experiences and understanding.

There can be no substitute for effective training, risk assessment and correct application of these. Human factors previously mentioned could also factor in, but ultimately personal, public and patient safety must prevail. Regulations are designed to guide, support, assess, teach and protect, and subject to the HASAWA (1974), healthcare professionals and their employers cannot ignore their duty of care to patients and visitors as well as to themselves, Health and Safety Executive (2024).

Case Scenario: A Hoist Lifting Incident

Working in a care home many years ago, colleagues were using a hoist to help transfer and move a patient. She weighed more than 90kg and had a limb amputation. There was a special sling to be used for her. Unfortunately, it was soiled and only a standard sling was available, but she was desperate to use the facilities. Staff felt there was no choice but to use the standard sling.

Despite their training, these experienced staff chose to carry out the task. In their efforts to mitigate risk and reduce risk of harm they chose to put the brakes on the hoist. This goes against training and procedural protocol for use of a hoist when lifting and moving a person.

While performing the manoeuvre, the hoist tipped over, and the patient and staff panicked.

The result:

Thankfully the patient was still hovering over the bed so landed on the bed. Staff quickly kicked the breaks off, released the emergency lever lowering the patient.

Unfortunately, staff and patient all suffered minor injuries and the patient feared going on a hoist for a long time after.

Staff were retrained, a spare sling was ordered, and it took weeks to work with the patient to regain her trust.

Everyone involved was lucky that their injuries were minor; it could have been much worse with la sting and life-changing injuries.

Conclusion

There is no doubt that clinical governance plays a pivotal role in the maintenance of a safe environment or improvement of quality of patient care. Risk assessment and risk management are at the heart of the process and with the primary objective of keeping patients safe. It is inevitable that due to human factors any given process may be flawed. Patients' harm may mean adverse or irreversible causes; nevertheless, it is important for healthcare staff to learn from mishaps. The mitigating factor should be the reporting of safety concerns as well as learning from any shortcomings when things go wrong. When this happens, lessons should be learnt to reduce the likelihood of the recurrence of any future harm.

Healthcare providers as employers have a duty of care to ensure the safety of all who come on their subject to section 2 (1) (e) of the HASAWA (1974, s 2(1) (e)). This includes patients, staff and visitors. Healthcare professionals likewise have a duty of care under section 7 of the HASAWA (1974), to ensure the safety of patients and that of others.

References

Berwick Report (2013) Available online at: https://www.gov.uk/government/publications/berwick-review-into-patient-safety

Birt J (2023) 5 whys technique: Root cause analysis (with examples). Available online at: https://www.indeed.com/career-advice/career-development/5-whys-example (accessed on 10th January, 2024)

Britannica (2024) Available online at: https://www.britannica.com/topic/bystander-effect (accessed on 3rd January 2024)

Bromiley Case. (2008). Available online at: https://publications.parliament.uk/pa/cm200708/cmselect/cmhealth/1137/1137we25.htm (accessed on 4th February 2024)

6Cs (no date) Available online at: https://www.nhsprofessionals.nhs.uk/nhs-staffing-pool-hub/working-in-healthcare/the-6-cs-of-care (accessed on 3rd January 2024)

Case Study (2017) Patient safety first: Reducing Harm from deterioration intervention – NHS Somerset 27 Project: To reduce the number of falls in community hospitals. Available online at: https://www.england.nhs.uk/wp-content/uploads/2013/11/nqb-hum-fact-concord.pdf (accessed on 21st February 2024)

CCF0010 – Evidence on NHS complaints and clinical failure. Available online at: https://committees.parliament.uk/writtenevidence/55955/html/#:~:text=The%20Swiss%20Cheese%20model%20as,number%20of%20layers%20of%20defences (accessed on 9th January 2024)

Coulter and Collins (2011) Liberating the NHS: No decision about me, without me. Available online at: https://assets.publishing.service.gov.uk/media/5a7c80cde5274a2674eab180/Liberating-the-NHS-No-decision-about-me-without-me-Government-response.pdf (accessed on 8th January 2024)

Citizen's Charter (1991) Available online at: https://publications.parliament.uk/pa/cm200708/cmselect/cmpubadm/411/41105.htm (accessed on 8th January 2024)

Department of Health (2008) High quality care for all: NHS next stage review final report (Lord Darzi Report). p47. Available online at: https://assets.publishing.service.gov.uk/media/5a7c3a5b40f0b67d0b11fbaf/7432.pdf (accessed on 6th January 2024)

Dyer C (2023, June 13) Police investigating dozens of patient deaths at hospital in Brighton. BMJ, 381, 1356. Available online at: https://www.bmj.com/content/381/bmj.p1356 (accessed on 22nd May 2024)

Fenn P, Diacon S, Gray A, Hodges R, Rickman N (2000 Jun 10) Current cost of medical negligence in NHS hospitals: Analysis of claims database. BMJ, 320(7249), 1567–1571.

Francis Freedom to Speak Up (2015). A review of whistleblowing in the NHS. Available online at: https://www.gov.uk/government/publications/sir-robert-francis-freedom-to-speak-up-review (accessed on 8th January 2024)

HASAWA 1974. s 2(1) (e) Available online at: https://www.legislation.gov.uk/ukpga/1974/37/contents (accessed on 22 May 2024)

HASAWA 1974. s 7 Available online at: https://www.legislation.gov.uk/ukpga/1974/37/contents (accessed on 22 May 2024)

Health Safety Executive (2024) Moving and handling in health and social care. Available online at: https://www.hse.gov.uk/healthservices/moving-handling.htm (accessed on 2nd February 2024)

Health and Social Care Act (2022) Available online at: https://www.legislation.gov.uk/ukpga/2022/31/contents/enacted

Healthcare Safety Investigation Branch (2023) Available online at: https://www.hssib.org.uk/ (accessed on 22nd January 2024)

HSE (1991) Introduction to human factors. Available online at: https://www.hse.gov.uk/humanfactors/introduction.htm (accessed on 9th January 2024)

Ishikawa K (1968) Guide to quality control. Tokyo, JUSE

Leadership Management and Quality (LMQ) Model (1993) Available online at: https://lmq.co.uk/aviation (accessed on 9th January 2024)

MHRA (2024) CAS. Available online at: https://www.cas.mhra.gov.uk/SearchAlerts.aspx (accessed on 23rd January 2024)

NHS Resolution (2020) Manual handling. Available online at: https://resolution.nhs.uk/resources/did-you-know-manual-handling/ (accessed on 20th January 2024)

NHS Resolution Performance Report and Accounts (2022/23) Available online at: https://resolution.nhs.uk/wp-content/uploads/2023/07/NHS-Resolution-Annual-report-and-accounts-2022_23-3.pdf (accessed on 5th January 2024)

NHS Serious Incident Framework (2015, 27 March) Investigations and complaints – Patient Safety Learning – the hub. Available online at: https://pslhub.org

NHS Serious Incident Framework (2015) Available online at: https://www.england.nhs.uk/wp-content/uploads/2015/04/serious-incidnt-framwrk-upd.pdf

NMC Code (2018) Available online at: https://www.nmc.org.uk/standards/code/

NPSA (2001) Available online at: https://www.npsa.org.uk/reporting/ (accessed on 8th January 2024)

Patient Safety Incident Response Framework (PSIRF) supporting guidance (2022, August) Engaging and involving patients, families and staff following a patient safety incident. Available online at: https://www.england.nhs.uk/wp-content/uploads/2022/08/B1465-2.-Engaging-and-involving…-v1-FINAL.pdf (accessed on 11th November 2023)

R v Letby Available online at: https://www.judiciary.uk/judgments/r-v-letby-2/

RCN Wheel (updated 2019) Available online at: https://www.rcn.org.uk/clinical-topics/Patient-safety-and-human-factors/Professional-Resources (accessed on 9th January 2024).

Reason J (1990) Human error. New York, NY, Cambridge University Press

Reason J (2013) A life in error: From little slips to big disasters. Farnham, Ashgate Publishing

Report of the Mid-Staffordshire NHS Foundation Trust Public Inquiry (Francis Report (2013) Available online at: https://assets.publishing.service.gov.uk/media/5a7ba0faed91 5d13110607c8/0947.pdf (accessed on 9th January 2024)

Reporting of Injuries, Diseases and Dangerous Occurrences Regulations (RIDDOR) (2013) available online at; https://www.hse.gov.uk/pubns/indg453.htm accessed on 9th January 2024.

Royal College of Radiologists (2019) Human factors | The Royal College of Radiologists. Available online at https://rcr.ac.uk

Safety Culture (2023) Available online at: https://safetyculture.com/topics/root-cause-analysis/ (accessed on 6th January 2024)

Serious Incident Framework (2014) Available online at: https://www.england.nhs.uk/wp-content/uploads/2015/04/serious-incidnt-framwrk-upd.pdf

Sign up to Safety (2014, updated in 2018)

The Health Foundation (1992) The health of the nation - A strategy for health in England white paper. Available online at: https://navigator.health.org.uk/theme/health-nation-strategy-health-england-white-paper (accessed on 4th January 2024)

WHO (2023) Patient safety. Available online at: https://www.who.int/news-room/fact-sheets/detail/patient-safety (accessed on 9th January 2024)

3 Equality, diversity, and inclusion in healthcare, does this happen?

If not, why not?

David Atkinson

Introduction – the right to health

The aim of this chapter is to identify the risks and dilemmas experienced by service users who are excluded or have difficulty in accessing their rights to healthcare due to their protected or other characteristics. It will include the Equality Act and the protected characteristics:

> Health is a state of complete physical, mental and social well-being and not merely the absence of disease or infirmity. The enjoyment of the highest attainable standard of health is one of the fundamental rights of every human being without distinction of race, religion, political belief, economic or social condition.
>
> WHO (2020)

> The right to health must be enjoyed without discrimination on the grounds of race, age, ethnicity, or any other factor. Non-discrimination and equality require states to take steps to redress any discriminatory law, practice, or policy.
>
> WHO (2022)

Equality

In general terms, equality is about opportunities for fair and putting everyone on a level playing field [Equality and Human Rights Commission (EHRC) 2018]. It is about ensuring that individuals, or groups of individuals, are not treated less favourably because of their protected characteristics (University of Edinburgh, 2022).

In healthcare the meaning is a little more specific as it is viewed as "treating people alike according to their needs" (Skills for Care, 2023).

Diversity

Simply described as 'The quality, condition, or fact of being diverse or different; difference, dissimilarity; divergence' (Oxford English Dictionary, no date);

DOI: 10.4324/9781003376934-3

however in healthcare, good diversity practice is ensuring that the services that are provided to people are accessible and fair to everyone involved irrespective of any protected characteristics or backgrounds. Both equality and diversity are essential components of health and social care. Good equality and diversity practices ensure that the services that are provided to people are accessible and fair to everyone involved, including service users and care providers.

Inclusion

Inclusive means "Including all types of people, things or ideas" (Cambridge Dictionary, no date) and treating them all fairly and equally. It means that all people, without exception, have the right to be included, respected, and appreciated as valuable members of the community.

'Inclusive health' is a 'catch-all' term used to describe people who are socially excluded, and who typically experience multiple overlapping risk factors for poor health (such as poverty, violence, and complex trauma), experience stigma and discrimination, and are not consistently accounted for in electronic records (such as healthcare databases). These experiences frequently lead to barriers in access to healthcare and extremely poor health outcomes. People belonging to inclusion health groups frequently suffer from multiple health issues, which can include mental and physical ill health and substance dependence issues. This leads to extremely poor health outcomes, often much worse than the general population, lower average age of death, and it contributes considerably to increasing health inequalities (GOV.UK, 2021).

Inclusion health includes any population group that is socially excluded. This can include people who experience homelessness, drug and alcohol dependence, vulnerable migrants, Gypsy, Roma, and Traveller communities, sex workers, people in contact with the justice system, and victims of modern slavery but can also include other socially excluded groups. There will be differences in needs within socially excluded groups (for example between men and women) and these differences must be understood and responded to appropriately (GOV.UK, 2021).

The law

In terms of the legislation, the overarching law is the 2010 Equality Act. Within the Act there are categories known as 'protected characteristics' (Equality Act, 2010), and these, among other real or perceived 'differences,' will be discussed further in this chapter. The Equality Act came into force in October 2010, and there are many sections and pages in the Act, but for the purpose of this chapter, the section on 'protected characteristics' is of paramount importance as many poor decisions, which sometimes also occur in healthcare, are based on misunderstanding or ignoring these elements of the Act. The Act brought together over 116 separate pieces of legislation, and it provides a discrimination law which protects individuals, and those with 'protected characteristics' from unfair treatment and "promotes a fair and more equal society" (EHRC, 2022). Discrimination may be direct or indirect.

In relation to healthcare practice, each characteristic will be discussed in turn, and for clarity and ease of reference they will be discussed in the order they appear in the Act, which does not indicate any order of preference or importance.

It is also important to note the relevance of Articles 2 The Right to Life, Article 3 Prohibition of Torture and Article 8 ECHR (1950) Right to Respect for private and family life, in the United Kingdom, this is applied by the Human Rights Act (1998).

Protected characteristics

These are age – by 2030, one in six people in the world will be aged 60 years or over (WHO, 2023) – disability, gender reassignment, marriage and civil partnership, pregnancy and maternity, race, religion or belief, sex, and sexual orientation, Equality Act 2010, ss.14 (1) and (2).

Age

Many older people are at risk of developing mental health conditions such as depression and anxiety disorders. Many may also experience reduced mobility, chronic pain, frailty, dementia, or other health problems, for which they require some form of long-term care. As people age, they are more likely to experience several conditions at the same time.

Whilst there are no known legal cases to date of age discrimination in healthcare, at least in the UK, this is due, at least in part, to the fact that following the publication of the Equality Act in 2010, in 2012 there was a ban in the National Health Service (NHS) on age discrimination in a healthcare setting (Dyer, 2012).

Thinking Point

However, there are situations that could involve age discrimination in a healthcare setting, for example, making assumptions about whether an older patient should be referred for treatment based solely on their age, rather than individual needs and level of fitness (Information Now, no date).

The United Nations Committee on Economic, Social and Cultural Rights stated in May 2000 "With regard to the realization of the right to health of older persons, the Committee, in accordance with paragraphs 34 and 35 of General Comment 1995, No 6, para 34 and 35, which reaffirms the importance of an integrated approach, combining elements of preventive, curative and rehabilitative health treatment. Such measures should be based on periodical check-ups for both sexes; physical as well as psychological rehabilitative measures aimed at maintaining the functionality and autonomy of older persons; and attention and care for chronically and terminally ill persons, sparing them avoidable pain and enabling them to die with dignity."

United Nations (2000)

It is worth noting that age discrimination does not necessarily mean it always occurs at the end stages of life, as according to Webb (2004), children also experience discrimination in healthcare and he posits that children, despite experiencing profound discrimination within society, are omitted from the general equality debate. He states that children experience significant discrimination, from both individuals and institutions. Such discrimination affects both their health and the quality and delivery of child health services (Webb, 2004). This is disturbing, not least because according to the Office for National Statistics (ONS), in 2019 the number of children in the UK (those aged under 16 years) increased by 8.0% to 12.7 million (ONS, 2021).

Thinking Point

A child aged 12 is experiencing distress at being in an Accident and Emergency reception area with adults waiting to see a doctor. What would you do?

1 Would you move them to another area or room; would you ignore this distress?
2 Is there anything else you could do to minimise their distress; would you prioritise this?

Disability

The latest estimates from the Department for Work and Pensions' Family Resources Survey indicate that 16.0 million people in the UK had a disability in the 2021/22 financial year. This represents 24% of the total population (UK Parliament, 2023).

A disability is a physical or mental impairment that has "a substantial and long-term negative effect on a person's ability to do normal daily activities. 'Substantial' means more than minor or trivial, for example taking much longer than it usually would to complete a daily task like getting dressed. 'Long term' means '12 months or more,' for example, a breathing condition that develops because of a lung infection" [GOV.UK, no date (a)].

The United Nations acknowledges a disabled person's right to both physical and mental health. It also raises awareness of the need for non-discriminatory practice when delivering healthcare. This applies to both public and private sectors (United Nations, 2000).

Case Scenario: Equality and Human Rights Commission (EHRC) v. a Clinical Commissioning Group (CCG)

The CCG had a policy limiting spending on continuing healthcare, which meant disabled people with ongoing health needs risked being moved from their homes into residential care against their wishes. EHRC believed this breached Human Rights Laws (Article 8 'Respect for your private life and family life, home and correspondence') and equality laws. Legal proceedings were commenced whereupon the CCG agreed to review their continuing healthcare policy, which will be monitored by the EHRC. The EHRC also wrote to 13 other CCGs advising them they were beginning Judicial Review proceedings for the same reasons. All of them accepted the failings of their continuing healthcare policies and agreed to revise them without the need for further legal action. The EHRC is continuing to monitor these CCGs to ensure they take the actions they have committed to (EHRC, no date).

Gender reassignment

The British Medical Association (BMA) cited data from the National Lesbian, Gay, Bisexual and Transgender (LGBT) survey (2018) which shows serious concerns, in that 40% of respondents who had accessed or tried to access public healthcare services reported having experienced at least one of a range of negative experiences because of their gender identity in the 12 months preceding the survey. In addition, 21% reported that their specific needs had been ignored or not considered, and 18% had avoided treatment for fear of a negative reaction.

The BMA commented that "Addressing these concerns is critical to providing high quality care and reducing health inequalities, as well as to ensure an inclusive healthcare system free from discrimination" (BMA, 2022).

Thinking Point

What would you do if you referred to a patient using the pronoun 'he' (as they are male in appearance) and they become angry and upset and insist on being referred to as 'she'?

This is known as misgendering and can make the person feel invalidated or disrespected, especially if it is done repeatedly or deliberately.

Marriage and civil partnership

Any discrimination experienced in this category may have been experienced by service users who had other protected characteristics, for example, sexual orientation and/or gender reassignment within same-sex marriages.

Case Scenario

A same-sex couple in a civil partnership are seeking advice about the health of their adopted child and are made to feel that they should not have children as they are both the same sex, despite identifying as having different genders.

Pregnancy and maternity

Service users with these protected characteristics do not, in of themselves experience discrimination; however, they may have other protected characteristics whilst being pregnant and during motherhood. For example, the MBRRACE (Mothers and Babies: Reducing Risk through Audit and Confidential Enquiries) Report (Birthrights, 2021) shows a disturbing disparity in maternal mortality rates between women from Black and Asian aggregated ethnic groups and white women, which is four times higher for Black women, and twice as high for mixed ethnicity women, and almost twice as high for Asian women. Amy Gibbs, CEO of Birthrights, stated, "We remain deeply concerned that Black and Brown peoples' basic human rights to safety, dignity and equality in pregnancy and childbirth are not being protected, respected or upheld" (Birthrights, 2021).

There is an ethnic group that is often missed in pregnancy and maternity discrimination discussions, and that is Gypsy, Roma, and Traveller communities, who were represented in May 2023 in Friends Families and Travellers (no date) (a national charity), in a published report on 'Maternal Health Inequalities in Gypsy Roma and Traveller Communities,' which in summary gave some disturbing information. There is a lack of awareness, sensitivity, and accommodation of cultural norms, such as those relating to maternity care, with stigma and taboo around perinatal mental health, as well as barriers to accessing mental health support. There are high rates of Caesarean birth reported by Gypsy, Roma, and Traveller research participants and consulted health professionals, and high rates of Classical Galactosemia among infants born to Irish Traveller parents, and high rates of miscarriage, pregnancy loss and/or child loss reported by Gypsy, Roma, and Traveller research participants. The report cited the UK Government as stating: "Gypsies, Travellers and Roma are among the most disadvantaged people in the country and have poor outcomes in key areas like health and education."

The recommendations in this report addressed each of the concerns raised, though the recommendations only went as far as stating what 'should' happen, rather than what 'must' happen, which seems to fall short of demanding what the Equality Act requires in terms of adherence to the law.

Thinking Point

Do you think laws such as the Equality Act 2010 should be more strictly enforced in cases like this?

Race

According to the UK 2021 census, 18% of the population belong to a Black, Asian, mixed, or other ethnic group [GOV.UK, no date (b)].

There are cases of racial discrimination against patients/service users, and there are numerous cases documented where racial discrimination is apparent in NHS staffing. In September 2022, the National Health Executive published an article about a survey demonstrating "worrying evidence of racial discrimination across a range of public institutions, including the NHS" (Morris, 2022). The results of this survey, which was commissioned by the Black Equity Organization, is the largest ever opinion poll of Black people detailing their experiences of living in Britain and showed that 65% of Black people had been discriminated against by healthcare professionals because of their ethnicity. The report also revealed the lack of confidence people had that change was coming, with 60% of Black respondents saying they did not see the changes necessary to address their experiences coming from the relevant institutions. In May 2023, the Kings Fund published an updated 'explainer' (originally published in February 2021 and updated September 2021) by Raleigh (2021) entitled "The health of people from ethnic minority groups in England." The publication is detailed and covers a broad range of ethnic minority groups and several health conditions. This publication highlights the need for further investigation into why these disparities occur and what needs to be done to eradicate these differences (Kings Fund, 2023).

In addition to the more obvious racial and ethnic groups in the UK, there is an ethnic group that often seems to be missed when racial discrimination is discussed and that is the Gypsy, Roma, and Traveller communities, which, according to the UK government, is a term used to describe people from a range of ethnicities who face similar challenges (GOV.UK, 2022). The report states that "Health outcomes for Gypsy, Roma, and Traveller communities are very poor compared to other ethnic groups." There is a lack of effective communication and accessible information in health services, and barriers to accessing and maintaining continuity of care, and barriers to accessing mental health support for Gypsy, Roma, and Traveller communities, with wider determinants of health, such as chronic shortages of Gypsy and Traveller sites, and insecure housing experienced by some members of the Roma community. There is discrimination, both direct and structural, within public services in healthcare and beyond, along with fear and mistrust of public services and state bodies (UK Parliament, 2019).

Some of these problems stem from living on Traveller sites or travelling, whilst others "stem from direct or indirect discrimination." There are problems registering and accessing General Practitioner (GP) services, immunisation services, maternity care, and mental health provision. Although some Clinical Commissioning Groups (CCG) and NHS Trusts show excellent practice in catering for the needs of this group, there is "evidence of widespread non-inclusion and in some cases, outright discrimination." In a prior report, McFadden (2019) outlined ways in which health services can exclude Gypsy, Roma, and Traveller patients, stating "There are subtle and not so subtle ways that people are restricted from registering with GPs. Sometimes it is not having the right paperwork and documentation, or not understanding what is required for proof of address, or simply not being able to provide it. There have been cases where a surgery had asked to see a bank statement prior to registration" (UK Parliament, 2019).

The government paper gives details of a range of services where these communities felt they received less than satisfactory healthcare services (GOV.UK, 2022).

Religion or belief

The 1948 UN Declaration of Human Rights makes it clear:

Article 1

All human beings are born free and equal in dignity and rights. They are endowed with reason and conscience and should act towards one another in a spirit of brotherhood.

Article 18

Everyone has the right to freedom of thought, conscience, and religion; this right includes freedom to change his religion or belief, and freedom, either alone or in community with others and in public or private to manifest his religion or belief in teaching, practice, worship, and observance. This right is also extended to atheists, as they have the right to choose not to follow any religion. This right also includes political opinion (Indirect, no date).

The WHO goes further in support of the European Convention on Human Rights 1950 and the Human Rights Act 1998. The definition of discrimination is very broad. This means that a victim may claim discrimination on the grounds which include the nine protected characteristics (Equality Act, 2010). Healthcare and wellbeing are included if a person is discriminated on the grounds of age or gender.

Swihart et al. (2023) published a very comprehensive article on cultural religious competence in clinical practice which detailed the large number of differences in 21 religions which would need to be considered when caring for anyone of these faiths. They go on to say that religious beliefs often affect patient attitudes and behaviour, and therefore it is important for healthcare professionals to understand these issues, so they can provide culturally appropriate care. It is equally important to remember that preservation of life overrides guidelines; in a life-threatening situation, there are usually no restrictions on medications or surgical interventions. However, when caring for a patient, it is important to understand why adherence or non-adherence to treatment may occur given their religious beliefs, and not to judge or discriminate due to these differences, and to acknowledge their right to choose their faith, and ask what could be done to care for them in the most appropriate way.

Sex

Liu and DiPietro Mager (2016) published an article in the United States about the importance of considering the differences between males and females in clinical decision making. They suggested that there are disease states which disproportionally or differentially affect women and went on to say that diseases which disproportionally affect women indicate a disease burden that is greater in women than in men. They gave examples which included breast cancer and urinary incontinence. They stated that diseases may also present differently in men and women, for example, women with cardiovascular disease may experience differences in signs or symptoms. They went further and identified the recognition of the need to include women sufficiently in clinical trials, though in previous decades the consideration and inclusion of men overshadowed women in clinical research design and conduct. This was observed when studying diseases prevalent in both sexes, where males, frequently of the Caucasian race, were the 'norm' study population. A type of observer bias, male bias, in assuming a male's attitude in conducting trials was another contributing factor. At the same time, researchers often thought that women would have the same response as men from drugs in clinical trials. They also viewed women as confounding and more expensive test subjects because of their fluctuating hormone levels (Liu & DiPietro Mager, 2016).

In the UK, according to the 2021 Census, 'women and girls' made up 30.4 million (45.3%) of the population of England and Wales (GOV.UK, no date (c)). The UK Parliament stated that women experience discrimination in health outcomes (UK Parliament, 2021). They cite a study by Manual, a wellbeing platform for men, which found that in many countries, men are more likely to face greater health risks. However, the UK does not follow this trend. It was found to have the largest female health gap in the G20 group of countries, and the 12th largest globally. It would seem from several sources of evidence that women are and have been discriminated against in healthcare across the world, and this discrimination includes clinical and pharmaceutical trials, and actual treatment of diseases and conditions. In her book 'Invisible Women,' Perez (2019) devotes two chapters to the lack of consideration of the differences between males and females in several ways, some of which could lead to fatal consequences if ignored. The causes of health inequalities or disparities are complex but are generally associated with variation in a range of factors that positively or negatively influence our ability to be healthy. This includes individual health-related behaviour, such as:

- smoking and diet
- access to services
- social deprivation
- access to work
- education levels
- social networks

(GOV.UK, 2021)

Perez (2019) includes many examples regarding the exclusion of women from trials and subsequent treatments, but from a UK perspective her research indicates some shocking evidence. For example, UK research indicates that women are 50% more likely to be misdiagnosed following a heart attack, partly due to women not having the 'Hollywood heart attack' (chest and arm pains), and may present without any chest pain, but with stomach pain, breathlessness, nausea, and fatigue. This is of particular concern as the National Institute for Clinical Excellence (NICE) (2014) guidelines specify unexpected acute chest pain as part of the criteria for a patient being referred for primary percutaneous coronary interventions (PPCI) at one of the specialist centres.

Perez (2019) further suggests that there are many conditions and diseases where diagnostic tests and checklists have been developed for boys and men, while girls and women present differently, such as in autism, which was previously thought to be more prevalent in boys, but recent research suggests there are far more girls with autism than previously realised. This seems to be due to differences in female socialisation, which may help girls mask their symptoms better than boys, but of course, male-orientated tests and checklists would not identify that difference. Similarly, early clinical research on attention deficit hyperactivity disorder (ADHD) and Asperger's syndrome was conducted on hyperactive white boys whereas girls presented as less hyperactive and more as disorganised, scattered, and introverted. Even conditions that by their very nature are 'women's problems' are ignored or denied. For example, premenstrual syndrome (PMS), which can include mood swings, anxiety, bloating, headaches, stomach pain, and sleep problems and affects

90% of women. It is under studied, with only a small range of medicines available, and as a result 40% of women do not respond to those medications (Perez, 2019). This is very disturbing as in extreme cases women have tried to kill themselves, yet despite this, researchers are being turned down for research grants on the basis that "PMS does not actually exist" (Perez, 2019, p. 373). Dysmenorrhea or period pains similarly affects up to 90% of women yet there is little that can be done as treatment options are limited. In 2013, sildenafil citrate (Viagra) was found to provide "total pain relief for over four consecutive hours with no observed adverse effects." This was discovered whilst the drug was being evaluated as a heart disease medication. It was not particularly successful at that, but when the trial participants (who were all male) reported an increase in erections, the researchers were more than keen to explore this newfound alternative use. Sadly, the trial had to be stopped because funding ran out, but what if the trial had included women? The doctor who led the study has applied twice for funding to compare sildenafil to the standard of care (a non-steroidal anti-inflammatory) but was rejected both times on the grounds that the reviewers "did not see dysmenorrhea as a priority public health issue," despite it affecting up to 90% of women. To highlight this disparity between the sexes, the US Food and Drug Administration approved the medical abortion pill after four years, in comparison with Japan, where the Ministry of Health took 35 years to approve oral contraceptive pills. In contrast, both the US and Japan registered sildenafil for erectile dysfunction in six months to ensure that the product reached men promptly (Ravindran et al., 2020).

Perez provides many other examples that clearly demonstrate "bodies, symptoms and diseases that affect half the world's population are being dismissed, disbelieved and ignored" (Perez, 2019, p. 234).

The United Nations recommended in 2000 that states integrate a gender perspective in their health-related policies, planning, programmes, and research to promote better health for both women and men. A gender-based approach plays a significant role in influencing the health of men and women. The separation of health and socio-economic data according to sex is essential for identifying and remedying inequalities in health and reducing risk, as to use a 'one size fits all' approach does not consider the obvious differences in the health needs of males and females as discussed above by Perez (2019). They added that to eliminate discrimination against women, there is a need to develop and implement a comprehensive national strategy for promoting women's right to health throughout their life span. This should include interventions aimed at the prevention and treatment of diseases affecting women, as well as policies to provide access to a full range of high quality and affordable health care, including sexual and reproductive services. A major goal should be reducing women's health risks, particularly lowering rates of maternal mortality and protecting women from domestic violence. The realisation of women's right to health requires the removal of all barriers interfering with access to health services, education, and information. It is also important to undertake preventive, promotive, and remedial action to shield women from the impact of harmful traditional cultural practices and norms that deny them their full reproductive rights.

Over 20 years later, the guidance from the United Nations and the World Health Organization is being ignored, as is the Equality Act, and as a result, women are suffering and dying, and this must stop.

Thinking Point

1   Were you aware that women's health and treatment is often based on tests and clinical trials with only male participants?
2   What are the ethical considerations?

Sexual orientation

According to NHS England (2017) "the evidence that LGBT+ people have disproportionately worse health outcomes and experiences of healthcare is both compelling and consistent. With almost every measure we look at LGBT+ communities fare worse than others. This is unacceptable, and we need to increase our efforts to address these health inequalities."

NHS England (2017) showed that in a survey, with over 108,000 responses, a situation where LGBT+ communities faced discrimination and felt their specific needs were not being met, had poorer experience and had major concerns about accessing healthcare that should be a right for all. The survey provides more details about their experiences, such as at least 16% of survey respondents who accessed or tried to access public health services had a negative experience because of their sexual orientation, and at least 38% had a negative experience because of their gender identity. Over half (51%) of survey respondents who accessed or tried to access mental health services said they had to wait too long, with 27% stating they were worried, anxious, or embarrassed about going and 16% said their GP was not supportive.

A large percentage (80%) of trans respondents who accessed or tried to access gender identity clinics said it was not easy, with long waiting times the most common barrier (NHS England, 2017). These findings prompted the formulation and publication of the LGBT Action Plan in 2018, which contained a number of proposals designed to improve access to healthcare and reduce or eradicate any discrimination felt or experienced by members of the LGBT community when doing so, and included the following recommendations: a National Adviser will be appointed to lead improvements to LGBT healthcare, and they will focus on reducing the health inequalities that LGBT people face and advise on ways to improve the care LGBT people receive when accessing the NHS and public health services. This would include working across the NHS to ensure that the needs of LGBT people are considered throughout the health system and will help towards improving healthcare professionals' awareness of LGBT issues so they can provide better patient care. The Adviser will work with relevant statutory organisations and professional associations to embed LGBT issues into physical and mental health services, and the NHS will improve the way gender identity services work for transgender adults.

The Government Equalities Office (2018) plan is expected to provide advice about the Gender Recognition Act (2004) for GP surgeries and gender identity clinics, along with improvements in the understanding of the impacts on children and adolescents of changing their gender and will gather evidence on the issues faced by people assigned female at birth who transition in adolescence, and action will be taken to improve mental healthcare for LGBT people. The Health Education England suicide prevention competency framework will cover high-risk groups including LGBT people. The National Adviser will work to ensure healthcare professionals understand the benefits of asking patients about their sexual orientation and gender identity, and action will be taken to improve the support for LGBT people with learning disabilities. The Department of Health and Social Care will review, collate, and disseminate existing best practice guidance and advice regarding LGBT issues and learning disability, and will also ensure that training requirements for support staff and advocates who work with people with learning disabilities includes advice regarding LGBT people (Government Equalities Office, 2018).

It remains to be seen whether these proposals are effective and continuing to evolve according to the needs of the LGBT community, as the NHS and Equality and Diversity Council is 'currently dormant' and there appears to be no other organisation or department within the NHS to address these issues.

Refugees and asylum seekers

There is one group worthy of inclusion, despite the fact they do not have a 'protected characteristic,' and this group are refugees and asylum seekers. This group has always been in existence, but in these days of increasing conflict and oppression in many countries, the number is steadily rising, and their needs are not to be ignored. In all four nations of the UK, refugees and asylum seekers with an active application or appeal are fully entitled to free NHS care. The situation for refused asylum seekers is more complicated and is not the same across all nations. According to the BMA, there is no evidence that refugees and asylum seekers use a disproportionate share of NHS resources, and migrants in the UK and elsewhere in Europe tend to use fewer services than native populations. However, they go on to say that refugees and asylum seekers in the UK often have difficulty accessing healthcare and other public services. In many cases, this could be because they may be unfamiliar with the way these services are organised or if there are documentation requirements.

Thinking Point

A refugee is in the GP surgery trying to register but has no documentation and is refused due to this fact. Is this correct? Do they need any documents to access healthcare?

The answer is no, as according to the BMA (2023), GP practices do not need to request any identity documents to register a new patient. However, some surgeries may ask patients to provide documents, including identification, proof of address and sometimes proof of immigration status in order to register. Any such requests must be non-discriminatory. For example, they cannot be based on the applicant's race, gender, social class, age, religion, sexual orientation, appearance, disability, or medical condition. This is clearly enabling inclusion based on the same criteria as anyone else in the UK, and it important to note that if a patient is not able to provide identity documents, it is not reasonable grounds to refuse to register them. In addition, refugees and asylum seekers are sometimes incorrectly denied or charged for secondary care because of confusion about their entitlement to NHS care. A BMA survey found that 55% of doctors who work with refugees and asylum seekers were frequently or sometimes uncertain about their entitlement to care. Female refugees and asylum seekers may have complex pregnancies, especially if they have experienced female genital mutilation (FGM) or other forms of violence. It is important that they receive proper medical support throughout their pregnancies. Unfortunately, confusion about entitlement to care means that many women are afraid of being charged or turned away and do not engage with maternity services. All maternity services are considered 'immediately necessary' and must never be delayed or refused (BMA, 2023).

Thinking Point

1   Have you experienced or are aware of any discrimination regarding any of the above protected characteristics in any healthcare setting?
2   Was anything done about it?
3   What would you do if you to encounter any discrimination in your place of work?
4   Is there anyone you could contact in your organisation?

Conclusion

As a final word, it is of concern that in response to an enquiry made in October 2023 to the Equality and Diversity Council at NHS England the reply was as follows:

> The NHS Equality and Diversity Council is currently dormant. Unfortunately, at this time we are unable to advise when the Council will be reconvened.

It would appear from this response that equality and diversity is not sufficiently important enough for government ministers or senior leadership in the NHS to employ anyone to deal with the issues involved. It would also appear that laws such as the Equality Act (2010) and the Human Rights Act (1998) are being ignored. This is extremely unfortunate as it would appear from the information in this chapter that most of the discrimination and lack of inclusion in all areas of healthcare is down to a lack of knowledge and understanding, and access to information and support for patients, service users, and staff alike would go a long way in eradicating these shortfalls in healthcare provision.

References

Birthrights (2021) Available online at: https://www.birthrights.org.uk/2021/11/11/new-mbr-race-report-shows-black-women-still-four-times-more-likely-to-die-in-pregnancy-and-childbirth/ (Accessed on 3rd November 2023)

British Medical Association (2022) Available online at: https://www.bma.org.uk/advice-and-support/equality-and-diversity-guidance/lgbtplus-equality-in-medicine/inclusive-care-of-trans-and-non-binary-patients#:~:text=Addressing%20these%20concerns%20is%20critical,healthcare%20needs%20as%20other%20patients (Accessed on 3rd November 2023)

British Medical Association (2023) Available online at: https://www.bma.org.uk/advice-and-support/ethics/refugees-overseas-visitors-and-vulnerable-migrants/refugee-and-asylum-seeker-patient-health-toolkit/overcoming-barriers-to-refugees-and-asylum-seekers-accessing-care (Accessed on 3rd November 2023)

British Medical Association (2023) Available online at: https://www.bma.org.uk/advice-and-support/ethics/refugees-overseas-visitors-and-vulnerable-migrants/access-to-healthcare-for-overseas-visitors/non-urgent-urgent-and-immediately-necessary-treatment-of-overseas-visitors (Accessed on 3rd November 2023)

Cambridge Dictionary (no date) Available online at: https://dictionary.cambridge.org/dictionary/english/inclusive (Accessed on 3rd November 2023)

Dyer C (2012) Age discrimination in UK healthcare will become unlawful in October. Available online at: https://www.bmj.com/content/344/bmj.e4134 (Accessed on 3rd November 2023)

Encyclopaedia Britannica (no date) Available online at: https://www.britannica.com/dictionary/eb/qa/difference-divergence-diversity (Accessed on 21st May 2024)

Equality Act (2010) Available online at: https://www.legislation.gov.uk/ukpga/2010/15/contents (Accessed on 21st May 2024)

Equality and Human Rights Commission (no date) Available online at: https://legal.equalityhumanrights.com/en/case/protecting-right-disabled-people-stay-their-own-home-1 (Accessed on 3rd November 2023)

Equality and Human Rights Commission (2022) Available online at: https://www.equalityhumanrights.com/ehrc-publishes-annual-report-and-accounts-2022-23 (Accessed on 6th November 2023)

European Convention on Human Rights (1950) Available online at: https://www.equalityhumanrights.com/sites/default/files/is-britain-fairer-accessible.pdf

Friends Families and Travellers (no date) Available online at: https://www.gypsy-traveller.org/wp-content/uploads/2023/07/Extended-Maternal-Health-Inequalities-Guidance.pdf, p 12 (Accessed on 3rd November 2023)

Government Equalities Office (2018) Available online at: LGBT Action Plan (https://assets.publishing.service.gov.uk/media/654e5fae8a2ed4000d720d0e/Great_Britain_Equality_and_Human_Rights_Monitor_Final_PDF.pdf) https://www.legislation.gov.uk/ukpga/2004/7/contents (Accessed on 3rd November 2023)

GOV.UK (2021) Available online at (Inclusion Health: Applying All Our Health – GOV.UK) www.gov.uk (Accessed on 3rd November 2023)

GOV.UK (2022) Available online at: https://www.ethnicity-facts-figures.service.gov.uk/summaries/gypsy-roma-irish-traveller (Accessed on 2nd November 2023)

GOV.UK (no date a) Available online at: https://www.gov.uk/definition-of-disability-under-equality-act-2010 (Accessed on 3rd November 2023)

GOV.UK (no date b) Available online at: https://www.ethnicity-facts-figures.service.gov.uk/#:~:text=Government%20data%20about%20the%20UK's,group%20(2021%20Census%20data (Accessed on 4th November 2023)

GOV.UK (no date c) Available online at: https://www.ethnicity-facts-figures.service.gov.uk/uk-population-by-ethnicity/demographics/male-and-female-populations/latest#:~:text=The%20data%20shows%20that%3A,up%2029.2%20million%20(49.0%25 (Accessed on 4th November 2023)

Human Rights Act (1998) Available online at: https://www.legislation.gov.uk/ukpga/1998/42/contents (accessed on 21st May 2024)

Health disparities and inequalities and health: Applying All our Health (2021) Available online at: https://www.gov.uk/government/publications/health-disparities-and-health-inequalities-applying-all-our-health/health-disparities-and-health-inequalities-applying-all-our-health (Accessed on 22nd May 2024)

Information Now (no date) Available online at: https://www.informationnow.org.uk/article/age-discrimination/# (Accessed on 4th November 2023)

Kings Fund (2023) Available online at: https://www.kingsfund.org.uk/publications/health-people-ethnic-minority-groups-england (Accessed on 3rd November 2023)

Liu KA, DiPietro Mager NA (2016) National Library of Medicine. Available online at: https://www.ncbi.nlm.nih.gov/pmc/articles/PMC4800017/ (Accessed on 12th December 2023)

McFadden A (2019) Available online at: https://publications.parliament.uk/pa/cm201719/cmselect/cmwomeq/360/full-report.html (Accessed on 3rd November 2023)

Morris L (2022) NHS providers publish anti-racism statement. Available online at: https://www.nationalhealthexecutive.com/articles/nhs-providers-publish-anti-racism-statement (Accessed on 3rd November 2023)

National Institute for Clinical Excellence (2014) Available online at: https://www.nice.org.uk/guidance/qs68/chapter/Introduction (Accessed on 3rd November 2023)

NHS England (2017) Available online at: https://www.england.nhs.uk/about/equality/equality-hub/patient-equalities-programme/lgbt-health/ (Accessed on 4th November 2023)

nidirect (no date) Available online at: https://www.nidirect.gov.uk/articles/religious-belief-and-political-opinion-discrimination#:~:text=Direct%20discrimination,philosophical%20belief%20or%20political%20opinion (Accessed on 12th December 2023)

Office for National Statistics CENSUS (2021) Available online at: https://www.ons.gov.uk/peoplepopulationandcommunity/populationandmigration/populationestimates/bulletins/annualmidyearpopulationestimates/mid2019estimates#:~:text=the%20number%20of%20children%20(those,by%2022.9%25%20to%2012.4%20million (Accessed on 4th November 2023)

Oxford English Dictionary (no date) Available online at: https://www.oed.com/search/dictionary/?scope=Entries&q=diversity (Accessed on 3rd November 2023)

Perez CR (2019). *Invisible Women: Exposing data bias in a world designed for men.* Penguin, London.

Raleigh V (2021). The health of people from ethnic minority groups in England. Available online at: https://www.kingsfund.org.uk/publications/health-people-ethnic-minority-groups-england) (Accessed on 3rd November 2023)

Ravindran TKS, Teerawattananon Y, Tannenbaum C, Vijayasingham L (2020). Making pharmaceutical research and regulation work for women. *British Medical*

Journal; 371:m3808. Available online at: https://www.bmj.com/content/371/bmj.m3808 (Accessed on 12th December 2023)

Skills for Care (2023) Available online at: https://www.skillsforcare.org.uk/resources/documents/Developing-your-workforce/Care-Certificate/Care-Certificate-Standards/Standard-4.pdf (Accessed on 3rd November 2023)

Swihart DL, Yarrarapu SNS, Martin RL (2023) *Cultural religious competence in clinical practice*. Available online at: https://www.ncbi.nlm.nih.gov/books/NBK493216/#__NBK493216_ai__ (Accessed on 3rd November 2023)

UK Parliament (2019) Available online at: https://publications.parliament.uk/pa/cm201719/cmselect/cmwomeq/360/full-report.html#heading-10 (Accessed on 3rd November 2023)

UK Parliament (2021) Available online at: https://lordslibrary.parliament.uk/womens-health-outcomes-is-there-a-gender-gap/ (Accessed on 3rd November 2023)

UK Parliament (2023) Available online at: https://commonslibrary.parliament.uk/research-briefings/cbp-9602/#:~:text=How%20many%20people%20have%20a,24%25%20of%20the%20total%20population

United Nations (2000) Available online at: https://digitallibrary.un.org/record/425041?ln=en (Accessed on 4th November 2023)

University of Edinburgh (2022) Available online at: https://www.ph.ed.ac.uk/equality-diversity-and-inclusion/about-edi/what-does-equality-diversity-and-inclusion-mean (Accessed on 3rd November 2023)

Webb E (2004) Discrimination against children. *Archives of Disease in Childhood*; 89:804–808. Available online at: https://adc.bmj.com/content/89/9/804.info (Accessed on 3rd November 2023)

World Health Organization (2020) Forty-ninth edition Including amendments adopted (in 2019) [Basic Documents]. https://apps.who.int/gb/bd/pdf_files/BD_49th-en.pdf#page=6

World Health Organization (2022) Available online at: https://www.who.int/news-room/fact-sheets/detail/human-rights-and-health (Accessed on 3rd November 2023)

World Health Organization (2023) Available online at: https://www.who.int/news-room/fact-sheets/detail/mental-health-of-older-adults (Accessed on 3rd November 2023)

4 Patient safety and accountability, civil and criminal law liability

Paul Buka

Introduction

The focus is on accountability in health and safety setting as applicable to the Civil – Tort law (or Delict – Scots Law) and Criminal Law branches. In a close caring relationship, liabilities are more likely to arise. The standard of care and patient safety matters, and governance (Chapter 2) can be achieved by working in partnership with the patient (NHS Constitution, 2012, updated 2018). Paternalism should no longer be the norm. The patient-staff relationship is fiduciary, i.e., based on trust. Due to dependence, vulnerable service users or patients may be at risk. The latter are now becoming more autonomous and informed of their rights. There is no guarantee to safety as things may go wrong, with patients being harmed. If this happens, the question is who should be held to account. Individuals should take responsibility for their actions or decisions, both positive and negative. This and key concepts will be explored further this chapter.

Setting the scene: Background

Accountability (2023) is defined as:

> The quality or state of being accountable especially, an obligation or willingness to accept responsibility or to account for one's actions.
> (https://www.merriam-webster.com/dictionary/accountability)

In a broader sense, accountability is related to formal settings where responsibilities, duties or expectations of a role are defined. However, in its broadest terms there are arenas of accountability which are linked to other formal settings (not necessarily work-related). For healthcare professionals, this will include professional accountability. This term is very broad and sometimes equated to responsibilities and 'duties' related to formal settings. On the other hand, the term 'liability' is more commonly applied to legal or financial/assets contexts.

Liability is:

> One of the most significant words in the field of law, liability means legal responsibility for one's acts or omissions. Failure of a person or entity to meet

DOI: 10.4324/9781003376934-4

that responsibility leaves him/her/it open to a lawsuit for any resulting damages or a court order to perform (as in a breach of contract or violation of statute.

Liability also applies to alleged criminal acts in which the defendant may be responsible for his/her acts which constitute a crime, thus making him/her subject to conviction and punishment.

(https://dictionary.law.com/Default.aspx?selected=1151#:~:
text=liability,for%20one's%20ac ts%20or%20omissions)

Clinicians should be covered by their professional indemnity insurance, and the employers' liability, provided they are acting in the line of duty, i.e., following local policy or guidelines/instructions.

In order to meet the objectives of the National Health Service Act (1946) and the NHS Constitution (2012), while maintaining safety, it was necessary to regulate an increasingly challenging area. This is in order to maintain and improve quality and protection of vulnerable patients who may be at the receiving end. Litigation USA-style is on the increase, and this can impact resources.

The World Health Organization (WHO) emerged in 1948 under the umbrella of the United Nations (UN), following the Second World War. The main aim was health promotion in order to keep patients safe. This presented a rather broad remit however in the interest of safe delivery of healthcare to service users, and this is paramount especially for care of vulnerable people. Advice of the WHO has a global impact on member countries, which should comply. There is no doubt that WHO policies shape international strategies including the United Kingdom's. One example is the more recent introduction of pandemics-related advice during COVID providing research and evidence-based guidance.

The WHO defines patient safety as follows:

Patient Safety is a health care discipline that emerged with the evolving complexity in health care systems and the resulting rise of patient harm in health care facilities. It aims to prevent and reduce risks, errors and harm that occur to patients during provision of health care. A cornerstone of the discipline is continuous improvement based on learning from errors and adverse events.

(WHO, 2019, https://www.who.int/news-room/
fact-sheets/detail/patient-safety)

Patient safety is fundamental to governance and delivery of quality and essential health services. Nevertheless, advances in medical science now continue to pose even greater challenges. This means that, as more people are living longer, with more complex health and social care needs, there will be both physical and psychological challenges. According to the Office of National Statistics (ONS, 2019), "…the population of the UK is ageing, and it is projected to continue to do so; by 2050, one in four people in the UK will be aged 65 years or over". Increasingly, it is clear that this will present even more challenges for healthcare providers and clinicians, who are expected to face them and to maintain high standards of care due to higher expectations. Due to limited resources, there is now a need for improving efficiency including reducing length of stay. This has also pressurised the services, with the potential danger of putting vulnerable service users at risk through early discharges or poor community care support.

Ongoing developments in healthcare technology should mean enhancing clinical governance and improving the quality of care. However, this may have its own problems associated with limited resources and increased demands. It is a challenge to maintain quality and standards. Although technology means enhanced standards, there is also risk regardless of how minimum it may be. The question is what level of risk can ever be 'acceptable'?

When human errors occur, mistakes are acknowledged, and apologies offered, this may go some way towards reparation for the victim. Defensive medicine on the other hand may encourage litigation.

After the inception of the NHS by the Labour government, by the then Minister of Health Aneurin Bevan in 1945, he acknowledged then that he expected some shortcomings.

Case Resource: NHS 1948 Inception and Patient Safety

'On 5th July we start together, the new National Health Service. It has not had an altogether trouble-free gestation! There have been understandable anxieties, inevitable in so great and novel an undertaking. Nor will there be overnight any miraculous removal of our more serious shortages of nurses and others and of modern replanned buildings and equipment. But the sooner we start, the sooner we can try together to see to these things and to secure the improvements we all want. My job is to give you all the facilities, resources and help I can, and then to leave you alone as professional men and women to use your skill and judgement without hindrance. Let us try to develop that partnership from now on'.

(Message to the medical profession, Bevan 1948, https://www.nuffieldtrust.org.uk/chapter/1948-1957-establishing-the-national-health-service#fn-1)

The Health and Safety Executive (HSE) was established on the 1 January 1975, with John Locke as its first director. Its main purpose was to enact the requirements of the Health and Safety Commission with the remit of enforcing the health and safety legislation. Key legislation was the Health and Safety at Work Act (HASAWA, 1974), except for workplaces which are regulated by Local Authorities. The HASAWA (1974) is an overarching regulatory responsibility for the health and safety of UK citizens. In the event of any safety breaches, the NHS, like other bodies, is subject to scrutiny by the HSE. The HSE is responsible for the inspection and prosecution of offenders. It also regulates, by formulating national guidelines and providing advice and updates of safety issues as well as national statistics. The HSE corroborates with the Care Quality Commission (CQC).

More recently, the appointment of the Patients Commissioner in June 2022 means that service users should have improved access in order to raise concerns. The Cumberlege Report (2020), Introduction to 'First Do no Harm', acknowledged the shortfalls within the recommended creation of a Patient Safety Commissioner position.

> The system is not good enough at spotting trends in practice and outcomes that give rise to safety concerns. Listening to patients is pivotal to that. This is why one of our principal recommendations is the appointment of an independent Patient Safety Commissioner, a person of standing who sits outside the healthcare system, accountable to Parliament through the Health and Social Care Select Committee. The Commissioner would be the patients' port of call, listener, and advocate, who holds the system to account, monitors trend, encourages, and requires the system to act. This person would be the golden thread, tying the disjointed system together in the interests of those who matter most.
>
> (Baroness Julia Cumberlege, Introduction to First Do No Harm, the Independent Medicines and Medical Devices Safety Review report 2020)

Bioethics, a legal framework for safety

Ethics and, more specifically, bioethics lays the foundation of the principle, 'duty of care', in order to ensure that the 'To do no harm' principle is applicable to and underpins safety. There were several versions of classical schools of thought in the branch of philosophy which was originally called Moral Philosophy or ethics of Socrates (470–399 BC), Plato (427/428–348/347 BC) and Aristotle (384–322 BC), but what they have in common are key principles of ethics comprising the first three of what is now the Bioethical framework or 'Bioethics', as adopted by Beauchamp and Childress (2019), as follows:

1 beneficence,
2 non-maleficence,
3 respect for autonomy and
4 justice, though the term 'Fairness' is preferable.

This framework has been at the heart of healthcare professional ethics since the publication of their first book in 1979. This has now been coined as 'the Principles of Biomedical (and healthcare) ethics – so called Principlism. Beauchamp and Childress (1979) have been credited with this more focused approach to ethics with application of ethics better structured than codes such as the largely obsolete Hippocratic Oath, which was traditionally taken by doctors (this was the attributed to Hippocrates (460–370 BC). Bioethics or Principlism has been since adopted by multidisciplinary teams for healthcare professionals and is at the heart of these core ethical principles. Encompassing safety is the 'To do no harm' principle which defines 'Beneficence' and 'Non-maleficence'. This is linked to the health and safety of vulnerable people as applied in HASAWA (1974). The term is generally applicable to advocating safety for potential victims. Some ethical theories are however associated with moral good and pleasure. One such example is the version of Utilitarianism, which stated that "fundamental axiom" that "it is the greatest happiness of the greatest number that is the measure of right and wrong", and "the obligation to minister to general happiness, was an obligation paramount to and inclusive of every other" [Bentham 1776 (1977, 393, 440)]. There is no correlation to patient safety.

Could the above Utilitarian principle be a factor in consideration of safety, in light of limited resources, the rights of the majority having pre-eminence over those of the minority? The ethics or morality of a given society pre-exists and informs the law. The latter may be informed by the former and not *vice versa*.

Primary legislation such as the HASAWA (1974), is passed by parliament. Delegated legislation, on the other hand, includes health and safety regulations which are passed by government departments and government bodies such as the HSE. The courts interpret and apply relevant law as they reach decisions, based on statutory interpretation and case law. The Scottish case, Donoghue v Stevenson (1932) *UKHL 100* (below) in the landmark case which introduced the 'neighbour principle' is applicable to health and safety.

Accountability and professional responsibility applied

Accountability is:

the quality or state of being accountable, especially,

an obligation or willingness to accept responsibility or to account for one's actions.

(https://www.merriam-webster.com/dictionary/accountability)

This concept is applicable within an ethico-legal framework.

Key: HASAWA 1974

Section 2. General duties of employers to their employees.

1 It shall be the duty of every employer to ensure, so far as is reasonably practicable, the health, safety and welfare at work of all his employees.
2 the provision and maintenance of a working environment for his employees that is, so far as is reasonably practicable, safe, without risks to health, and adequate as regards facilities and arrangements for their welfare at work.

Section 7. General duties of employees at work.
It shall be the duty of every employee while at work –

a to take reasonable care for the health and safety of himself and of other persons who may be affected by his acts or omissions at work.

(https://www.legislation.gov.uk/ukpga/1974/37/section/7#:~:text=7%20General%20 duties%20of%20employees,U.K.&text=(b)as%20regards%20any%20duty,be%20 performed%20or%20complied%20with)

There is a need for healthcare professionals to be held to account by their employer, professional bodies and the patient. Health and Safety law is applicable in both Civil and Criminal Law (this will be applied below). As discussed at the beginning, the term accountability is associated with but is different in application to 'liability' when it comes to criminal law compensation (via damages for negligence) thus making good to the victim of loss or harm such as pain and suffering. Ethical or moral values should be the basis of human actions; however, it may be difficult with limited effectiveness or remedy or real consequences as they may be based on societal or peer pressure. This is when the law steps in.

Human rights law is the vehicle for prosecution of breach of human rights breaches (as defined by the European Convention for Human Rights (ECHR 1950)). This was enacted by 14 articles in the Human Rights Act 1998. Human rights actions may be pursued directly in UK courts. Accountability and liability in Health and Safety case falls under the duty of care in Civil or Criminal Law.

Case Scenario: Accountability and Liability

Mr. U, in his early 80s diagnosed with mild dementia, living on his own in sheltered accommodation was admitted to hospital via A & E having sustained a suspected compound fracture of his right leg, lateral malleolus following a suspected high impact fall at home. He was found by his son who he had phoned soon after as he was lucky to have his house phone close by. The surgeons operated, with internal fixation of a pin and plate he was discharged five days, post-surgery. The surgeons left no specific instructions in the patient notes, on post-discharge care. The ward had also apparently forgotten to refer the patient to District Nurse (DN) for after care, wound dressing and monitoring. Dressings were not changed for three days, when the community physiotherapist noticed that the patient was complaining of pain, and seeing the swollen leg, urgently called the DN, who, on subsequently changing the dressing, noticed early signs of gangrene.

The patient is now facing potential septicaemia and possible amputation.

Thinking Point

1   Who should be held to account for the catalogue of errors?
2   What recommendations would you make so this does not happen again?
3   Please apply accountability in Tort, Criminal Law and Professional accountability.

Accountability is also relevant in the professional context. Healthcare professionals are registered with and subscribe to a regulatory body's code of profession conduct. This means that they must practise their ethical code of professional conduct. The healthcare professional codes of conduct are aligned to the bioethical principles as well as the above-mentioned safety legislation HASAWA (1974). Failure to comply will mean that, if reported, a healthcare professional may face a fitness to practice hearing, which is not directly related to an employment disciplinary hearing. The latter may mean imposition of sanctions or striking off conditions of practice or they may have no case to answer. If they are convicted of a crime, it is likely that an automatic referral to the professional body of registration fitness to practice hearing will follow.

The CQC England and Care Inspectorate (Scotland) took responsibility (from the National Patients Safety Agency) for patient or service user health and safety since April 2015. This applied to healthcare providers registered with them; HSE had enforcement responsibility, hence its investigation and subsequent prosecution.

The CQC set Fundamental Standards related to safety:

> You must not be given unsafe care or treatment or be put at risk of harm that could be avoided. Providers must assess the risks to your health and safety during any care or treatment and make sure their staff have the qualifications, competence, skills and experience to keep you safe.
>
> (CQC Fundamental Standards4 2022,
> https://www.cqc.org.uk/about-us/fundamental-standards)

Human rights in the UK were introduced in UK legislation since the country became signatory to the ECHR 1950. Article 3 (above) is key, as it relates to patient safety, as follows: 'No one shall be subjected to torture or to inhuman or degrading treatment or punishment'.

In clinical practice, especially mental health or learning disability, human rights challenges may arise for staff responding to potential complaints related to detention or seclusion and restraint, which are provided for patients under compulsory admissions subject to sections 2–5 of the Mental Health Act 1983.

Duty of care, civil liability

The following case forms the foundation of the duty of care concept and civil liability in Tort or Delict (Scots Law).

Case Law: Donoghue v Stevenson (1932) UKHL 100

On 26 August 1928, Mrs Donoghue's friend bought her a ginger-beer from Wellmeadow Café [1] in Paisley. She consumed about half of the bottle, which was made of dark opaque glass, when the remainder of the contents was poured into a tumbler. At this point, the decomposed remains of a snail floated out causing her alleged shock and severe gastro-enteritis.

Mrs Donoghue was not able to claim through breach of warranty of a contract: she was not party to any contract. Therefore, she issued proceedings against Stevenson, the manufacture, which snaked its way up to the House of Lords.

She was awarded damages on the basis of 'duty of case' or 'the neighbour principle'.

(https://www.lawteacher.net/cases/donoghue-v-stevenson.php)

The principle developed by Lord Atkin in the above case established when a duty of care might arise.

... is that one must take reasonable care to avoid acts or omissions that could reasonably be foreseen as likely to injure one's neighbour. A neighbour was identified as someone who was so closely and directly affected by the act that one ought to have them in contemplation as being so affected when directing one's mind to the acts or omissions in question.

(Donoghue v Stevenson 1932, AC 562 (HL Sc)
(Snail in the Bottle case))

Accountability in civil law sets a lower standard and burden of proof for successful litigation, on a balance of probabilities. Any person injured as a result of a health and safety breach may also bring a civil action in compensation for personal injury alongside criminal prosecution. Falling under Civil Law, remedies is accountability for the regulatory healthcare professional codes of conduct, which also requires the lower (civil) bar. Professional bodies may discipline registrants following complaints or referrals by employers or the public, with sanctions (there may also be criminal liability where intent or 'gross negligent manslaughter').

Duty of care is part of accountability and Clinical Governance and quality of care. Breach of legal standards of care may have implications on other branches of the law, such as criminal. Accountability in Tort law or Delict (Scotland) (Negligence) includes patient safety and is based on the duty of care as established in the famous Donoghue v Stevenson (1932) *UKHL 100* (above). This was a case on grounds of civil liability re: a victim of negligence by a manufacturer of ginger beer which contained the remains of a decomposed snail. The principle in the above landmark case has been applied to cases of clinical negligence, Lord Atkins 'neighbour principle' approach in his judgement, '...people must take reasonable care not to injure others who could foreseeably be affected by their action or inaction'. This became known as the 'subjective test' as it is based on the defendant's perspective, or 'contemplation'. Such an approach, however, could be fraught with difficulties of interpretation should a respondent/defendant contest accountability or liability for harm. This is the basis for compensation in Tort or law of negligence.

Tort Law, however, developed some clarity on the subjective test by substituting it with the 'objective test' in a subsequent case, Caparo Industries plc v Dickman(1990) *2 AC 605 House of Lords* (below). Lord Bridge revisited the process of establishing duty of care and accountability and highlighted the 'neighbour principle' and what was known as the 'objective test'; this is based on the reasonable man (or person) test. This now means that the court must look beyond the subjective perception of 'foreseeable harm' by a defendant. The new test (of duty of care) must be 'objective'.

Case Law: Caparo Industries Plc v Dickman [1990] 2 AC 605 House of Lords

Caparo Industries purchased shares in Fidelity Plc in reliance of the accounts which stated that the company had made a pre-tax profit of £1.3M. In fact, it turned out that Fidelity had made a loss of more than £400,000. Caparo brought an action against the auditors claiming they were negligent in certifying the accounts.

Held: That there was no duty of care owed in this case due to a lack of proximity between Caparo Industries and the auditors. This was due to the reason that since the auditors were not aware of 'the existence of Caparo nor the purpose for which the accounts were being used by them'.

(Lord Bridge (The Caparo test), https://e-lawresources.co.uk/cases/Caparo-Industries-v-Dickman.php)

In the above case, Lord Bridge clarified the 'neighbour principle' (which was established in the Donoghue case, please see the facts above). Accordingly, the right of an injured plaintiff or party to claim damages (or compensation) must now also be based on the 'neighbour principle' or 'closeness' between the plaintiff (injured party) and defendant (person being sued or their employers). Such closeness is not difficult to establish in a clinical relationship which is fiduciary, i.e., based on trust.

The court may award compensation or damages for personal injury, depending on the nature and severity. The harm or injury suffered may include psychological harm as well as loss of future earnings. A victim of clinical negligence may have a successful claim in Tort/Delict Law (law of negligence); this does not exclude from a Health and Safety Award though this may be taken into consideration in the event of a successful personal injury action. The standard of proof is on a balance of probabilities. Any award is in compensation for the harm suffered. The objective of the court is to put the victim in the position they would have been, had the harm not taken place. A victim of clinical negligence claiming damages for personal injury will most likely include the following headings:

Compensation for damages in medical negligence are categorised into two, namely:

1 General damages – Compensation for physical injury, pain and suffering, psychological injury and 'loss of amenity'
2 Special damages – compensation for any past and future financial losses for which causation (negligence) has been established.

(https://www.medicalnegligencedirect.com/
claiming-damages-for-clinical-negligence/)

Additionally, the NHS can now recover damages from a third party, such as an insurer following a Road Traffic Accident, under the NHS Injury Cost Recovery Scheme with a cap of £57,892 per injury.

Duty of care and criminal liability

Criminal law relates to intent, and the prosecution must prove the defendant's *mens rea* (guilty mind) linked to a guilty action, *actus reus*. This requires a higher standard of proof, which must be 'beyond reasonable doubt'. The burden of proof is on whether a perpetrator committed the misdemeanour 'with malice aforethought' or recklessly as in gross negligence manslaughter cases such as the Adomako case (see below).

Professional accountability means that a criminal prosecution may follow in relation to not only offences, for example, minor assault or petty theft, but could also escalate to more serious ones such as sexual offences, manslaughter or murder. Acts of 'wilful neglect' or recklessness may be a precursor of gross negligence manslaughter. The principle of accountability or liability in criminal law suggests a higher standard of evidence (of proof) than in civil cases as discussed above. It is necessary to prove a *mens rea* or intent, sometimes called 'a guilty mind'. The burden of proof lies on the prosecution and should be beyond reasonable doubt or in case of recklessness as to the outcome of one's actions. One example is a case of gross negligence manslaughter, which is established on 'recklessness' – the fact that a defendant was aware of and considered the consequences but, nevertheless, could not care less and went ahead. Suspected criminal cases must be reported to the police who should investigate and, with evidence of a crime, may charge any suspects who will be referred to the Crown Prosecution Service. In cases of suspected serious crimes occurring within clinical settings, charges may arise under Offences against the Person Act 1861, which includes murder or manslaughter, see the R v Adomako (1994) *3 WLR 288* below.

Case Law: R v Adomako (1994) 3 WLR 288

The appellant was an anaesthetist in charge of a patient during an eye operation. During the operation an oxygen pipe became disconnected, and the patient died. The appellant failed to monitor or notice or respond to obvious signs of disconnection.

- Imagine you are on the jury.
- What verdict would you return and why?

Verdict,

- The jury convicted Adomako of gross negligence manslaughter.

The Court of Appeal dismissed his appeal on the following grounds that,
"…in cases of manslaughter by criminal negligence involving a breach of duty, it is a sufficient direction to the jury to adopt the gross negligence test" (Lord Mackay of Clashfern LC on page 187).

The HSE or Local Authority may also bring a criminal prosecution against service providers. It is important to note that a breach of health and safety laws in one case may attract both civil and criminal law sanctions. The HASAWA (1974) applies to a variety of settings where there are human factors and activities. This includes any environment (including healthcare) which may be public or private buildings and facilities such as transport, leisure and the workplace. Any person may report a suspected breach to the HSE. Offending healthcare providers may also be criminally liable and prosecuted by the HSE, with imposition of fines and compensation may also be awarded to the victim or their representatives. The sanction may be either a fine, imprisonment or both. There may also be a case for corporate manslaughter.

The prosecutable category includes any criminal actions, and this applies to all healthcare staff such as doctors, nurses, physiotherapists, psychotherapists, paramedics as well as ancillary healthcare workers such as healthcare assistants and porters who may be employed by a healthcare provider.

The case of R v Turbill and Broadway (2014) *1 Cr.App.R. 7l* (below) defined the law and the criminal law standard of evidence (beyond reasonable doubt) into statute law. Following this case, the criminal law standard of proof is now enshrined in statute, as the Criminal Justice and Courts Act (CJCA, 2015).

Section 21(5) CJCA 2015 is intended to avoid a care provider escaping liability by relying on some alleged illegality on the part of the victim or an argument that the victim had in some way consented to a risk of harm when consenting to care or treatment.

Section 21(6) CJCA 2015 provides that a breach of duty is "gross" if the conduct alleged falls far below what can be reasonably expected of the care provider in the circumstances.

The issue in point is a requirement for the prosecution to prove intent of wilful neglect (by a healthcare provider or employee) in respect of a service user. At times more than one arena of accountability may be applicable. The following case includes civil, criminal liabilities as well as professional accountability. Depending on the circumstances with evidence of a systems failure, another category of criminal charge may follow under the corporate manslaughter heading.

Case Law: In R v Turbill and Broadway (2014) 1 Cr.App.R.7, Judgment: Hallett LJ

Four members of staff at a care home in Bromsgrove were charged with wilful neglect of one of their residents, contrary to s44 of the Mental Capacity Act (2005). The resident was Mr Thomas Milroy, an elderly man, suffering from Alzheimer's disease, osteoarthritis and hypertension. He was disorientated in time and place; he could not always recognise his children and his biological clock was confused. There was a note on his care plan to the effect that he was 'a high-risk faller'. His condition was obviously declining.

The Court applied the meaning of "wilful neglect" as set out in Sheppard to an offence contrary to section 44 of the Mental Capacity Act 2005. The Court stated that the term "wilfully" means deliberately refraining from acting or refraining from acting because of not caring whether action was required or not.

(https://vlex.co.uk/vid/r-v-maxine-turbill-805796597)

Thinking Point

1 Are you aware of the whistleblowing policy in your organisation?
2 Do you agree that employers should be prosecuted for corporate manslaughter?

Healthcare providers' senior management may now be investigated for corporate manslaughter subject to the Corporate Homicide Act 2007, which introduced a new offence for prosecuting organisations in cases proved to have a gross failure in health management and safety with fatal consequences. There have been calls for this more recently in the case of Letby, who killed seven babies and attempted to kill another seven. Letby was sentenced on Monday, 21 August 2023, and received a whole life order (x14), without parole. The judge said that she '... showed malevolence bordering on sadism'. She was the fourth woman in British history to be given a whole life order. A public enquiry has been announced by the government. Alternatively, an employer may be prosecuted subject to section 2 or 3 of the HASAWA (1974) where the evidence points to breach of duty of care but limited evidence of a systemic failure. Manslaughter may be classified as voluntary where there is intent, or involuntary, which may be described as 'negligent' and 'reckless'.

Consider the example below.

Case Study: Defendant: Cwm Taf Morgannwg University Health Board

On 13th November 2019, the patient absconded from Llynfi Ward, Maesteg Community Hospital through an unsecured ward main door. Approximately 10 minutes later, on entering the bay, the registered nurse was alerted to the patient being absent. As a result, staff on duty began a search of the Outpatients Department, the rear and front of the building. The patient called out in response to a member of staff who was calling their name. She was found on the floor at the bottom of seven steps located directly outside the hospital main entrance doors. The registered nurse reports that she assessed the patient prior to moving her, for limb deformity. The only obvious injuries found at the time were a laceration to the back of her head which was bleeding and a graze to their left knee.

This case did result from the investigation of a fatality.

Offence Date 01/04/2019

Total Fine   £800,000.00

Total Costs Awarded to HSE   £10,627.30

(https://resources.hse.gov.uk/convictions-history/defendant/defendant_details.asp?SF=DID&SV=4196945)

It is also useful to reflect on and apply the duty of care, which is defined in and applied to section 2 of the HASAWA (1974) and relates to the duties of the employer, which are based on the duty of care established in Donoghue v Stevenson (1932) UKHL 100. Furthermore, under section 7 of the HASAWA (1974), the same duty of care is also applicable to the employee, to ensure that no patient, healthcare professional or other person is harmed as a result of their negligence.

Case Study: Health Board Fined £180,000 After Patient Dies, 14 February 2023

Re: NHS Highland, of Assynt House, Beechwood Park, Inverness (2023) A health board was fined £180,000 after a patient died while being treated at a hospital. Colin Lloyd, 78, was brought to Raigmore Hospital, Inverness, on 6 February 2019 following a suspected fall at his home and later admitted to the hospital's surgical ward. While in hospital, Mr Lloyd suffered from three additional falls on 6, 12 and 14 February 2019, which led to bleeding in the brain. Mr Lloyd passed away from fatal head trauma two days after his final fall.

An investigation by the HSE found that NHS Highland, the health board responsible for Raigmore Hospital, failed to provide the necessary nursing staff to ensure the 1:1 ratio of care was applied. NHS Highland, of Assynt House, Beechwood Park, Inverness, pleaded guilty to breaching Regulation 5(1) of the Management of Health and Safety at Work Regulations 1999. The health board was fined £180,000 at Inverness Sheriff Court on 31 January 2023.

HSE (2023) inspector Penny Falconer said: "This incident could so easily have been avoided by simply carrying out correct control measures and safe working practices. Organisations should be aware that HSE will not hesitate to take appropriate enforcement action against those that fall below the required standards".

(https://press.hse.gov.uk/2023/02/14/health-board-fined-180000-after-patient-dies/?utm_source=govdelivery&utm_medium=email&utm_campaign=press-channels-push&utm_term=health-board-fine&utm_content=news-16-feb-23)

Thinking Point

1 Please identify crucial interventions in the patient's care plan, which would have minimised the risk of falls.

When things go wrong: Vicarious liability and indemnity

Due to human factors, and even with the best will in the world, things may go wrong when a patient is harmed due to a variety of reasons. Sadly, there may also be circumstances where a service user may be victim of clinical negligence. As seen above, a victim or injured party may claim damages for personal injury, and in some cases, a health and safety and/or criminal prosecution may ensue.

The Report of the Mid Staffordshire Foundation Trust Public Inquiry (2013) made some recommendations on learning from past errors with five key recommendations:

- A "common culture" has been proposed throughout the NHS.
- The report places emphasis on the creation of a "safety culture".
- An organisation should have shared values from top management to frontline staff.
- The NHS must have strong, consistent leadership to motivate staff.
- Everyone employed by the NHS should have a "questioning attitude, a rigorous approach and good communication skills".

(Report of Mid Staffordshire NHS Foundation, 2013, https://assets.
publishing.service.gov.uk/government/uploads/system/uploads/
attachment_data/file/279124/0947.pdf)

A key Francis Report (2013) recommendation was that healthcare providers and clinicians should learn from any errors in order to ensure that this does not happen again.

Being fair sets out the argument for organisations adopting a more reflective approach to learning from incidents and supporting staff. Whatever the culture, dealing with concerns about a professional's practice can be challenging.

(NHS Resolution, https://resolution.nhs.uk/resources/being-fair/)

In employment law, the notion of vicarious liability is based on the '*respondeat superior*' principle. This means that, as an employer benefits from the positive aspects of their employees' contributions and work, they hold responsibility for their employees' liabilities as long as the latter are following policy and guidelines. This principle however should be qualified. They should nevertheless also bear responsibility based on the assumption that the employer is in a stronger financial position, and it is not unusual for only them to be liable for prosecution and fined or be sued in litigation for damages in personal injury cases. However, in principle, the employees may also be sued under the principle of 'joint and several liability'. The employer is more likely to be sued because they are in a better position to have more resources. In practice, this is down to the taxpayer paying as the NHS healthcare providers are insured by the NHS Resolution to whom they pay an insurance premium.

The principle of the employer's vicarious liability arises when something goes wrong, though the employer may be in dispute if an employee was not following orders or policy or acting outside their remit, in which case they may be personally liable. Indemnity may cover them.

The law – The 'close connection test' means that a respondent person may be held accountable for the actions of another because of a special relationship the parties maintain, such as employer/employee. The close connection test will determine vicarious liability based on the type of contract, or if the respondent was acting in the course of their employment. At the heart of vicarious liability, the question arises whether a contract is of services or for services.

A contract of service is established on the principle that whoever determines the terms and conditions of employment and pays the wages must bear vicarious liability for their employees' actions [as likewise, they (employer) benefits from the positive actions of employees]. The principle established in law meant that an employer may be held to be vicariously liable for the actions (in Tort/Delict Law) due to the 'relative closeness' if an employee is acting in the course of their employment.

Case Law: The 'Close Connection' Test: Barclays Bank Plc v Various Claimants (2020) UKSC 13 (1 April 2020)

The Supreme Court has overturned a decision that a bank was vicariously liable to claimants suing in respect of alleged sexual assaults by a doctor carrying out pre-employment medical examinations.

The doctor was an independent contractor carrying out (mostly) pre-employment medical examinations for Barclays Bank, up to the mid-80s. He did so at his home where he had a consulting room, and the bank paid him a fee for each examination. Many of the bank recruits were females aged 15 or 16. The doctor died in 2009. He also did medical examinations for a different employer (a mining company) and an insurance company and carried out sessions at local hospitals.

Held: That the key question was whether the tortfeasor (the doctor) was carrying on business on his own account or whether he was in a relationship akin to employment with the defendant (the bank). Here the doctor was carrying on business on his own account. Therefore, the bank was not vicariously liable.

Thinking Point

1 Do you agree with the Supreme Court decision?
2 If the doctor had been still alive at the time of trial, what chances would the victims have had to sue personally for personal injury?
3 What key recommendation would you make to ensure this does not happen again in future?

As to the question of what happens to a clinician who chooses not to follow national guidelines and local policy, this means that the employer who is sued may in theory litigate, in turn, against such an employee, in order to recoup their losses. Professional indemnity insurance is now a requirement for professional registrants subscribing to bodies such as the Health and Care Professions Council (HCPC), Nursing and Midwifery Council (NMC) and General Medical Council (GMC). In all circumstances, the healthcare professional must always be able to justify their decisions and actions within healthcare.

Conclusion

If healthcare provision were based on ethics alone, it would not suffice for the purpose of ensuring patient safety. There is a need for providing patient safety, fairness and remedies for any breaches by healthcare providers and staff, who must be held to account.

The development and application of bioethics as a discipline had been linked to healthcare, specifically, the 'To do no harm' principle is relevant and should be at the heart of patient safety.

The law now is built on and supersedes ethical principles, which are the basis of accountability or liability in civil and criminal law. In today's litigious society, however, the link of the term 'accountability' to the Bioethical Principles is inevitable and appropriate. This means that the development of duty of care in Tort Law (Delict in Scotland) bodes well with the bioethical principle 'To do no harm'. This branch of law encompasses Tort (Delict) Criminal and health and safety laws. This area is also informed by ethics and the principle of 'accountability' or 'answerability' extending to the employer and employees. The question of duty of care is now embedded in UK law as well as Common Law and other Roman-Dutch influencing jurisdiction such as Scots Law. The principle is key to trust and fiduciary duty and is linked to the question of 'accountability' and 'liability' in the event of things going wrong at the heart of a breach of trust in healthcare provision.

References

Accountability (2023) Available online at: https://www.merriam-webster.com/dictionary/accountability (Accessed on 1st November 2023)

Barclays Bank plc v Various Claimants (2020) UKSC 13

Beauchamp TL, Childress JF (1979) *Principles of Biomedical Ethics.* New York: Oxford UP (Bioethics)

Beauchamp TL, Childress JF (2019) *Principles of Biomedical Ethic,* 8th ed. New York: Oxford UP (Bioethics)

Bentham J (1776 [1977, 393, 440n]). Available online at: https://plato.stanford.edu/entries/bentham/#:~:text=In%20the%20Fragment%20Bentham%20stated,1977%2C%20393%2C%20440n%5D (Accessed on 20th November 2023)

Bevan A (1948) Nuffield Foundation Available online at: https://www.nuffieldtrust.org.uk/chapter/1948-1957-establishing-the-national-health-service#fn-1 (Accessed on 20th November 2023)

Caparo Industries plc v Dickman (1990) 2 AC 6 Criminal Justice and Courts Act (CJCA, 2015).05 House of Lords

Corporate Manslaughter and Corporate Homicide Act (2007) Available online: https://www.
legislation.gov.uk/ukpga/2007/19/contents (Accessed on 23rd May 2024)

CQC Fundamental Standards (2022) Available online at: https://www.cqc.org.uk/about-us/
fundamental-standards (Accessed on 22nd May 2024)

Criminal Justice and Courts Act (CJCA, 2015) Available online at: https://www.legislation.
gov.uk/ukpga/2015/2/contents (Accessed on 22nd May 2024)

Cumberlege Report (2020) First do no harm, the independent medicines, and medical devices
safety review report. Available online at: https://www.hqip.org.uk/the-baroness-cumberlege-
report-first-do-no-harm-published-8th-july-2020/ (Accessed on 22nd May 2024)

Cwm Taf Morgannwg University Health Board. Available online at: https://resources.hse.
gov.uk/convictions-history/defendant/defendant_details.asp?SF=DID&SV=4196945
(Accessed on 19th November 2023)

Dictionary.Law.com. Available online at: https://dictionary.law.com/Default.aspx?
selected=1151#:~:text=liability,for%20one's%20acts%20or%20omissions (Accessed on
19th November 2023)

Donoghue v Stevenson (1932) UKHL 100

European Convention for Human Rights (ECHR 1950) Available online at: https://www.
coe.int/en/web/human-rights-convention/the-convention-in-1950#:~:text=The%20
Convention%20for%20the%20Protection,force%20on%203%20September%201953

Health and Safety at Work Act (HASAWA) (1974): s2 & 3, HASAWA (1974) and s7,
HASAWA (1974). Available online at: https://www.hse.gov.uk/legislation/hswa.htm
(Accessed on 222nd May 2024); https://www.legislation.gov.uk/ukpga/1974/37/
contents

HSE (2023) Available online at: https://press.hse.gov.uk/2023/02/14/health-board-fined-
180000-after-patient-dies/?utm_source=govdelivery&utm_medium=email&utm_
campaign=press-channels-push&utm_term=health-board-fine&utm_content=news-
16-feb-23 (Accessed on 20th November 2023)

HSE (2023, 14th February) Health board fined £180,000 after patient dies. Available
online at: https://press.hse.gov.uk/2023/02/14/health-board-fined-180000-after-pa-
tient-dies/?utm_source=govdelivery&utm_medium=email&utm_campaign=press-chan-
nels-push&utm_term=health-board-fine&utm_content=news-16-feb-23 (Accessed on
19th November 2023)

Human Rights Act (1998) Available online at: https://www.legislation.gov.uk/
ukpga/1998/42/contents (Accessed on 22nd May 2024)

Medical Negligence Direct. Available online at: https://www.medicalnegligencedirect.com/
claiming-damages-for-clinical-negligence/ (Accessed on 19th November 2023)

Mental Capacity Act (2005) Available online at: https://www.legislation.gov.uk/
ukpga/2005/9/contents (Accessed on 22nd May 2024)

Merriam-Webster. Available online at: https://www.merriam-webster.com/dictionary/
accountability (Accessed on 19th November 2023)

National Health Service Act (1946). Available online at: https://www.legislation.gov.uk/
ukpga/1983/20/contents (Accessed on 23nd May 2024)

NHS Constitution 2012, updated 2018

NHS Injury Cost Recovery Scheme (2023) Available online at: https://www.gov.uk/
government/publications/nhs-injury-cost-recovery-scheme (Accessed on 18th November
2023)

Office of National Statistics (2019) Available online at: https://www.ons.gov.uk/people-
populationandcommunity/populationandmigration/populationestimates/articles/overvie-
woftheukpopulation/august2019 (Accessed on 19th November 2023)

ONS (2020) Living longer and old-age dependency – what does the future hold? Available
online at: https://www.ons.gov.uk/peoplepopulationandcommunity/birthsdeathsandmarriages/
ageing/articles/livinglongerandoldagedependencywhatdoesthefuturehold/2019-06-24
(Accessed on 19th November 2023)

R v Adomako (1994) 3 WLR 288 house of lords

R v Turbill and Broadway (2014) 1 Cr.App.R. 7

Re: NHS Highland, of Assynt House, Beechwood Park, Inverness (2023) Available online at: https://press.hse.gov.uk/2023/02/14/health-board-fined-180000-after-patient-dies/?utm_source=govdelivery&utm_medium=email&utm_campaign=press-channels-push&utm_term=health-board-fine&utm_content=news-16-feb-23 (Accessed on 19th November 2023)

Report of Mid Staffordshire NHS Foundation (2013) Available online at: https://assets.publishing.service.gov.uk/government/uploads/system/uploads/attachment_data/file/279124/0947.pdf (Accessed on 19th November 2023)

s44, Mental Capacity Act (2005) Available online at: https://www.legislation.gov.uk/ukpga/2005/9/section/44 (Accessed on 22nd May, 2024)

ss2–5, Mental Health Act (1983). Available online at: https://www.legislation.gov.uk/ukpga/1983/20/contents (Accessed on 22nd May 2024)

World Health Organization (2019) Patient safety. Available online at: https://www.who.int/news-room/fact-sheets/detail/patient-safety (Accessed on 19th November 2023)

5 Treatment, therapies - medicines management and patient safety

Paul Buka

Introduction

The outcome of an appropriate patient assessment/examinations and investigations may lead to diagnosis, prescription and administration of medications. This process is part of medicines management, which is defined as 'the clinical, cost-effective and safe use of medicines to ensure patients get the maximum benefit from the medicines they need, while at the same time minimising potential harm' (DoH, 2004, p. 151).

'Treatment' includes all physical aspects in medicine, surgery and/or healthcare, nursing regimes, physiotherapy or speech therapy and psychological interventions. The aim should be to control or alleviate symptoms, pain and suffering and possibly cure. Medication management includes related therapies which may be physical, psychological or a combination of both. The multidisciplinary team should work in partnership in the treatment and medicines management.

Prescribing is the responsibility of suitably qualified healthcare professionals. The pharmacist dispenses medications, with frontline healthcare staff such as nurses, the patient themselves or their carers administering medications. Safe prescribing and administration of medicines should therefore be at the heart of healthcare provision in order to keep the patient safe.

The Health and Safety at Work Act (HASAWA, 1974) sections 2 and 7 define a duty of care for employers and employees (healthcare professionals), respectively, requiring risk assessments and risk management plans to be implemented (confer with Chapter 2 and 7). This is to minimise the likelihood of harm to patients. Individual care plans should be patient-centred and adapted to individual needs. Care pathways should be clearly defined and based on established protocol or tried-and-tested treatment strategies. Due to human factors, they may be inadequate, with resulting harm to patients due to system failures, drugs interactions or reactions. Unfortunately, clinical negligence or criminal actions may result in harm to patients. It is also possible that established treatment regimens or therapies may not always be effective or may be unfortunately ineffective or have adverse interactions.

DOI: 10.4324/9781003376934-5

Overview, medicines classification

The Medicines Act (1968) classified medicines into the following:

1 Prescription only (POMs), which could only be prescribed by a doctor and sup-plied by a pharmacist. This includes controlled drugs (CDs)
2 There would also be pharmacy (P) medicines which may be sold without a prescription.
3 General sales, which may be purchased from any shop with certain restrictions. (Examples included in 2 and 3, above, are painkillers).

Herbal medicines are not licenced. Under the Medicines Act (1968), which established an Independent Medicines Commission which reports to the Health Ministers of the UK (the licencing authority). In other words, it would be a crime to manufacture medicines without a licence. The Human Medicines Regulations (2012) consolidates the earlier statute, Medicines Act (1968), and is currently the primary legislation.

National policies which provide guidance on medicines prescription and admin-istration have derived from the legislative requirements of seminal statutes like the Medicines Act (1968) and the Human Medicines Regulations (2012), which con-solidated the former. Further guidelines are from the Royal Pharmaceutical Society (2013) Core Principles and the National Institute of Health and Care Excellence (NICE) 2015 Guidelines, which should be followed. Local policy and guidelines for individual healthcare providers should also embedded in the national policy (see Chapter 2).

Classification includes controlled drugs which are used in treatment, which nevertheless may also be illicit and addictive. These are subject to the Misuse of Drugs Act (1971) (as amended in 2010) 'to control use of powerful new narcotic drugs. This statute also aims to prevent misuse of controlled drugs by introducing a complete ban on possession, supply and manufacture as well as importing and exporting controlled drugs. The Misuse of Drugs Act (2005) regulates the use and storage of controlled drugs in clinical settings. Since 2019, cannabis-based medi-cines may now be prescribed for certain conditions such as 'intractable nausea and vomiting, chronic pain, spasticity and severe treatment resistant epilepsy'. Drugs controlled under the Misuse of Drugs Act (1971) are placed in 1–5 schedules to the Misuse of Drugs Regulations (2001), and they govern the import and safe storage of controlled drugs.

> The Statute also prohibits certain activities in relation to 'Controlled Drugs', in particular their manufacture, supply, and possession (except were permit-ted by the 2001 Regulations or under licence from the Secretary of State).
> (NICE, 2023, https://www.legislation.gov.uk/ukpga/1971/38)

Since the above 1971 Act, there has been new classifications of several con-trolled drugs, and some may appear to overlap, for example, in the case of some amphetamines. The BNF (2023) lists three main classifications of drugs as follows:

1   Class A, which includes methadone, morphine or fentanyl,
2   Class B, which includes oral amphetamines, dihydrocodeine tramadol and
3   Class C and this also includes certain categories of amphetamines like buprenorphine benzodiazepine, tramadol.

The above is in common use in clinical practice and therefore warrants serious attention from health professionals.

Clinical governance, medicines and extended prescribing

As early as 2000, there was a clinical governance drive towards improving the quality of care to enhance patient safety (confer with Chapter 2). This coincided with the introduction of non-medical prescribing, which aimed to ease the burden and workload of medical general practitioners (GPs) in the community. Clinical governance is at the heart of quality-of-care initiatives for patient-centred care (Scally and Donaldson, 1998). The Neighbourhood nursing: a focus for care (Cumberlege, 1986) Report had included a recommendation to allow community nurses and health visitors to prescribe medication as part of their work. This was also seen as a key aspect of the impetus towards improving quality of care. The Crown Report (1989) highlighted the excessive workloads for GP doctors. The primary legislation was the Medicinal Products: Prescription by Nurses etc. Act 1992, which provided for nurses to prescribe from a restricted list of drugs and application.

This was ground-breaking and resulted in a national programme of training, beginning in 1998, for all qualified district nurses and health visitors with community care nurses. This was also driven by the NHS Plan (2000), which aimed to provide 'a health service fit for the 21st century', and designed around the patient (patient centred), as a change framework for the Modernisation Agenda. This also facilitated the recommendation to extend non-medical prescribing as provided for by the Prescription by Nurses Act 1992 (above), which updated the Medicines Act (1968). Initially, this was limited to district nurses and health visitors, but subsequently incorporated other allied healthcare professionals who have undergone appropriate training.

Subsequently, Section 63 of the Health and Social Care Act (2001) provided for the expansion of prescribing responsibilities to other health professions. The extended role also now includes allied healthcare clinicians with three classifications of prescribers, Independent, Supplementary and Community Practitioner (Courtney Griffiths, 2010). A supplementary prescriber works with an independent prescriber while designing an agreed clinical management plan which should be implemented with the patient's permission. The scope of practice now extends to other healthcare professionals who have undertaken an appropriate programme of training which is validated by the Nursing and Midwifery Council and the Health Care Professional Council.

Independent prescribers (V300) can assess, diagnose and prescribe from the full British National Formulary, and supplementary prescribers (V300) can only prescribe in accordance with the clinical management plan. These two groups include the following healthcare professionals:

- *Nurses/midwives*
- *Pharmacists*
- *Physiotherapists*
- *Podiatrist*
- *Paramedics*
- *Optometrists*
- *Therapeutic radiographers and*
    Supplementary prescribers only
- *Diagnostic radiographers*
- *Dieticians*
    Community Practitioner Prescribers (V100 or V150 who are prescribers from a limited formula)
- *Nurses (health visitors and district nurses)*

(NHS Health England, 2023, hee.nhs.uk)

The Human Medicines Regulations (2012) provided for the production, import, distribution as well as the control of supply of medicines. This is part of pharmacovigilance, which is explored in the section below. The Medicines Health products Regulatory Authority (MHRA) is responsible for issuing the licence based on a successful clinical trial of a new drug or a known drug with a different use. Following the 'First do no harm', the Cumberlege Report (1986) recommended the creation of a new role of Patient Safety Commissioner (PSC) with the aim 'to promote patient safety in relation to medicines and medical devices and to promote patients' voices. The PSC role is in its developmental stage and is now also closely aligned with patient advocacy charities. It is hoped to provide an additional voice for vulnerable people at risk of harm.

Medicines administration: key pharmacological concepts

Polypharmacy ensues when patients are taking five or more medications for several medical conditions, resulting in possible interactions. Such individuals may be vulnerable and potentially at a higher level of risk, especially if they are taking a combination of medicines for several conditions. A prescriber should consider the fact that the more the number of prescribed medications, the higher the risk for the patient. Also, at risk are service users under the care of different specialities, due to possible conflicting or duplicate medications. The risk may be worsened by unprescribed over-the-counter or homeopathic remedies. An increase in medications may result in contraindication, interaction, overdosing and duplication or cancelling out the benefits of one drug. Groups who may be at a higher risk include individuals on complex medicines regimens and persons lacking capacity or those who are physically or psychologically frail. Polypharmacy is more likely to be associated with patients who have been subject to multiple admissions and may result in deterioration of health and/or fatal consequences, especially for so-called revolving-door patients. Key pharmacological concepts which are associated with risk for vulnerable patients will also be considered below.

Pharmacodynamics is a key concept which requires clinicians involved in the prescribing as well as the administration chain to take note of the possible adverse impact of medicines and how they work. This relates to the effect of a drug on the body, described as 'the study of a drug's molecular, biochemical, and physiologic effects or actions'. It comes from the Greek words *pharmakon*, meaning *drug*, and *dynamikos*, which means *power*. This process includes four stages: absorption, distribution, metabolism and excretion of the medication Marino et al. (2023). When considering the other side of the coin, pharmacokinetics (below) relates to the human body's reaction by accepting or rejecting a drug.

Pharmacokinetics, on the other hand, relates to passage of a drug, from absorption (route), distribution, metabolism and secretion (ADME) (Thomson, 2009). How drugs work varies from person to person, depending on factors affecting breakdown and absorption. Examples are age, gender, body weight, pathophysiology as well as drug interactions.

Pharmacogenetics, sometimes called pharmacogenomics, involves research-based tests related to drug responses based on individual genes for optimal selection of drug. This may help, for example, in the development of drugs for the effectiveness of treatment of a range of genetic conditions, such as cystic fibrosis. This model may be expensive and have ethical implications and therefore is less commonly used. It should be distinguished from ethnopharmacology, which is linked to pharmacological research, as a developmental discipline aiming to identify drugs for relieving human illness based on an analysis of previously unknown plants which may have been commonly in use to alleviate pain and suffering in some isolated cultures throughout the world. One example of such 'traditional' medication development was that of aspirin and morphine, which are derived from the bark of the willow tree.

Psychopharmacology relates to the scientific study and drugs which are used for treating mental health conditions and relates to prescription and administration of medications which are used for treating mental health disorders. It also considers the administration and impact of psychotropic medications which treat a variety of mental health-related conditions, and it carries its own risks. This may depend on individual pharmacokinetics (above). Examples are antidepressants, anti-anxiety or antipsychotics and mood stabilisers which will have some effect on the neurotransmitters in the brain. These drugs may pose similar risks to this group of patients due to the biopsychosocial nature of human beings. Similar to interactions, a contraindication may also result in an adverse drug reaction (ADRs). Risk is always present (for some patients) in the administration of psychotropic medicines.

Pharmacovigilance

While employers have a bioethical duty of care to ensure safety, under section 2 of HASAWA 1974, this also applies to clinicians, under section 7, to carry out an appropriate risk assessment and implement a risk management plan. They must evaluate the effectiveness and impact of any proposed interventions within the treatment regimen and medicines. They must also be vigilant and monitor the impact while working in partnership with the patient. This term also involves monitoring the effect and assessment in order to improve medicines' effectiveness in order to prevent drug complications (Waller, 2009). In the emergence of a pandemic, such monitoring has been re-defined as 'the science and activities relating to the detection, assessment, understanding and prevention of adverse effects or any other medicine/vaccine related problem' (WHO, 2020).

As part of health and safety, staff are required to assess risk with a management plan while monitoring the effect of medications, both positive and potentially hazardous. There is a need for thorough discharge planning in order to prevent 'revolving door patients'. This can happen if patient information on medications is not managed properly.

Duty of care and patient safety

A framework on procedures for prescribing and administration of medicines is based on duty of care *(Donoghue v Stevenson, 1932, UKHL 100)*.

Case Law: Donoghue v Stevenson (1932) UKHL 100

On 26 August 1928, Mrs Donoghue's friend bought her a ginger-beer from Wellmeadow Café [1] in Paisley. She consumed about half of the bottle, which was made of dark opaque glass, when the remainder of the contents was poured into a tumbler. At this point, the decomposed remains of a snail floated out causing her alleged shock and severe gastro-enteritis.

Mrs Donoghue was not able to claim through breach of warranty of a contract: she was not party to any contract. Therefore, she successfully issued proceedings against Stevenson, the manufacture, all the way up to the House of Lords.

(https://www.lawteacher.net/cases/donoghue-v-stevenson.php)

Thinking Point

1   Bioethics is based on four principles; can you name them?
2   Consider which one(s) apply directly to the 'to do no harm' principle?

The above case defined duty of care, underpinning minimising risk of harm to keep patients safe. It was estimated that there are 237 million medication errors in the NHS in England every year (Care Quality Commission, 2017). This is also enshrined in health and safety legislation as part of risk assessment and risk management. This applies the duty of care for the employer under section 2 and for employee under section 7 of the HASAWA (1974). Section 7 of the HASAWA 1974 requires the safety of patients and others who may be affected by their (healthcare staff's) actions or omissions. The Health and Safety Executive (HSE) provides a national framework (with a minimum requirement, based on a template form) for risk assessment. This is applicable to any setting where there are human activities which may put people at risk. It is important to follow a structured and logical progression in risk assessment:

* *Identify the hazards.*
* *Decide who might be harmed and how.*
* *Evaluate the risks and decide on precaution.*
* *Record your findings and implement them.*
* *Review your assessment and update if necessary.*

(HSE, http://www.hse.gov.uk/risk/fivesteps.htm)

It is not possible to guarantee elimination of all risks. The aim for clinicians should be to minimise risk to an acceptable level. The question arises then as to what level is 'acceptable'. The patient should be made aware of this fact when obtaining informed consent. Please reflect on the example below.

Case Study: Best Practice Guidance on the 'Safe Use of Oxygen Cylinders' to Help NHS Organisations Prevent Risks

During periods of extreme pressure, often exacerbated by a surge in respiratory conditions, the demand for oxygen cylinders, particularly small cylinders, increases in the NHS. This is due to the need to provide essential oxygen treatment in areas without access to medical gas pipeline systems. This surge in demand increases the known risks associated with the use of medical gas cylinders, and introduces new risks across three main areas:

* Patient safety
* Fire safety
* Physical safety

(NHS England, 2023b)

Thinking Point

Consider what risks could be posed to:

1 Patients
2 Staff members and visitors

As applied, medicinal products are 'intended for or, capable of performing, a medical function' [Medicines Healthcare products Regulatory Agency (MHRA), 2020]. This means that prescribers, pharmacists, dispensing staff and those who administer medicines directly, including doctors and nurses, family members and carers, all owe the patient a duty of care to ensure their (patient's) safety [Donoghue v Stevenson (1932) *AC 562* (above)]. The principle of concordance should be applied. This means that they (clinicians) must, if practicable, include the patient in the decision-making by obtaining informed consent. The likely source of risk is human factors related to unsafe systems and/or unsafe working practice, including human error which could be attributed to staff or patient errors. Additionally, ADRs (see next section) may follow.

The above principle applies to all medical procedures and requires a clinician and prescriber to obtain informed consent. Subject to the principle of 'concordance', they should discuss with the patient the treatment options as well as the benefits and detriments and potential side effects of the planned course of action. It may be difficult for a clinician to judge how much information is required by the patient. While capacity is a key element, informed consent (to treatment) must be obtained from the patient, with exceptions in emergencies or where the patient lacks capacity under the Mental Capacity Act (2005), in which case Deprivation of Liberty Safeguards (DoLS) may be applied. In the future, the updated Liberty Protection Safeguards (LPS) introduced in the Mental Capacity (Amendment) Act 2019 will be applied, the implementation date is awaited. Where applicable, patients may be sectioned and detained, with compulsory treatment subject to sections 2–5 of the Mental Health Act (1983). The question on how much information is sufficient is answered in the Montgomery case (below). In the absence of consent, a patient is entitled to recover damages for negligence if a clinician failed to diagnose their condition or gave an incorrect diagnosis, for errors during procedures and possibly administered the wrong drug or wrong dose. A prescriber must also offer alternative options as an obligation to warn the patient of potential risks of the proposed treatment. A patient is also entitled to know the likely consequence of refusing treatment.

Case Law: Montgomery (Appellant) v Lanarkshire Health Board (Respondent) [2015] UKSC 11

The above case drew attention to informed consent. Nadine Montgomery, a woman with diabetes and of small stature, delivered her son via the normal birth canal; she experienced complications owing to shoulder dystocia, resulting in hypoxic insult with consequent cerebral palsy. Her obstetrician had not disclosed the increased risk of this complication in vaginal delivery, despite Montgomery asking if the baby's size was a potential problem. Montgomery sued for negligence, arguing that if she had known of the increased risk, she would have requested a caesarean section.

The ruling overturned a previous decision by the House of Lords, which had been law (Bolam Test rejected).

Held

That, rather than being a matter for clinical judgment to be assessed by professional medical opinion, a patient should be told whatever they want to know, not what the doctor thinks they should be told.

It was accepted that shoulder dystocia can cause serious complications for mother and baby but also accepted that the risk of cerebral palsy was low, at around 0.1%.

Mrs Montgomery claimed for negligence, arguing she should have been told of all the risks.

She was awarded over £5 million in damages, after an appeal went to the Supreme Court.

Thinking Point

1 How much information is a sufficient degree?
2 What should happen is consent is obtained improperly?

An error in prescribing could result in a wrong prescription and administration of medicines. This may be due to a deficit in knowledge or due diligence, as well as possibly not following the correct procedure. Examples are route, incorrect dosages, frequency of administration, as well as the purpose for which the medication was prescribed. It is also possible to have the wrong combination of medicines, which could counteract each other. When dispensing, there is also a case for currency in use by dates or errors in Soundex, medicines which sound similar but are totally different. It is also possible for the patient to have an ADR.

The National Patient Safety Agency (NPSA, 2007) suggested that 71% of fatal and serious harm from medication incidents are errors due to human factors.

Mulac et al found that medication errors occurred during administration (68%) and prescribing (24%). The leading types of errors were dosing errors (38%), omissions (23%) and wrong drug (15%). The therapeutic areas most involved were analgesics, antibacterials and antithrombotic. Over half of all errors were harmful (62%), of which 5.2% caused severe harm, and 0.8% were fatal.

(Mulac et al., 2021)

All the above may result from human factors which are contributory to errors and patient harm. Healthcare providers and clinicians have a duty of care to ensure (as is humanly possible) safe prescribing, dispensing and administration of medicines and to ensure that no person is harmed because of their clinical negligent actions or omissions.

Clinicians must ensure a thorough approach to risk assessment and risk management, more so for medicines to minimise potential harm to patients. The Royal Pharmaceutical Society (2013) identifies the need for a key element of medicine management, which is the process of optimisation of medicines linked to 'a patient-centred approach'. This is also based on the Bioethical principles of doing good and avoiding harm. Utilitarianism could be applicable as safe administration of medicines does relate to outcomes and effectiveness use of medicines. The evaluation of the effectiveness of medications is important to check the optimisation of medicines. Concordance enhances working in partnership with the patient when obtaining informed consent to treatment, and this facilitates partnership between the clinician and patients. The ten Rs serve as a framework for minimising errors:

1 *Right patient*
2 *Right medication*
3 *Right dose*
4 *Right route*
5 *Right time*
6 *Right patient education*
7 *Right documentation*
8 *Right to refuse*
9 *Right assessment*
10 *Right evaluation, including monitoring the patient's response*

(Nursing Notes, 2015, 2018,
https://nursingnotes.co.uk/resources/10-rights-of-medication-administration/)

Case Law: Prendergast v Sam Dee Ltd and Others (1989)

A prescription was incorrectly dispensed by a community pharmacist who misread Amoxil as Daonil, which is an oral hypoglycaemic, and it caused unconsciousness and irreparable brain damage. The pharmacist argued that the error arose as a result of poor handwriting on the prescription. The court accepted that when writing a prescription there is a duty to write it legibly. The question for the Court of Appeal was how legible it must be.

The Court concluded that the writing of the word fell below the standard of legibility required in the exercise of a duty of care because it was written so as to invite or reasonably permit misreading under ordinary working conditions. The Court was satisfied that the prescriber's bad writing initiated a chain of events that led to harm. The consequence of writing a word which could reasonably be misread was to make it reasonably foreseeable that a different drug to the one intended might be dispensed to the patient.

Held: Pharmacist 75% liable for that harm: GP 25% liable for his poor handwriting

The Court of Appeal upheld judgement and added that there is a duty to write clearly so that busy or careless staff can read your instructions.

Thinking Point

What additional measures would you recommend in order to ensure safety in prescribing and administration of medicines, thus preventing this from happening again?

The Medicinal Healthcare Products Regulatory Agency (MHRA) was established in April 2003 following a merger of the Medicines Control Agency and the Medical Devices Agency. The MHRA is an executive govenrment agency (Department of Health), which has responsibility for ensuring the safety of medicines and medical devices. Complementary and Alternative Medicines (CAMs) include other forms of therapies which may be in use. The former may be used in conjunction with medicines, while the latter may be independent of medicinal treatment. The mental well-being aspects of treatment are important as they may work in conjunction of medications as well as psychological or talking therapies like cognitive behaviour therapy (CBT) for conditions such as anxiety. Other forms of psychological therapy include meditation, counselling and hypnotherapy. There are also physical aspects such as acupuncture or physiotherapy.

Incorporating CAMs was clearly a positive move in changing the nature of treatment, thus enhancing outcomes and holistic care. Complementary medicines may be taken alongside other conventional treatment. The problem however is that complementary medicines could counteract or cancel out the effects of prescribed conventional medicines.

'Health-related therapies' is a broad term encompassing physical or psychological aspects. This includes physiotherapy, acupuncture or mind-body related therapy such as cognitive behavior. This plays a key part in therapy. Other options of complementary therapies are also available. Complementary therapy is used in conjunction with or instead of conventional medicinal treatment. This may be used in conjunction with drug therapy.

Further examples of CAMs include:

- Nutritional (e.g., special diets, dietary supplements, herbs and probiotics)
- Psychological (e.g., mindfulness)
- Physical (e.g., massage, spinal manipulation)
- Combinations such as psychological and physical (e.g., yoga, tai chi, acupuncture, dance or art therapies) or psychological and nutritional (e.g., mindful eating)
(https://www.nccih.nih.gov/health/complementary-alternative-or-integrative-health-whats-in-a-name)

A few psychiatry hospitals are still using electric convulsive therapy (ECT) where indicated for adults, with exogenous or reactive depression. The success rate was moderate and '...in 2018-2019, 68% of people who had been treated with ECT were "much improved" or "very much improved" at the end of treatment' (Royal College of Psychiatrists, 2019). The use of drugs always carries a risk. It is a question of risk assessments and the benefits outweighing those risks.

Adverse drug reaction, near misses-yellow card reporting, black triangle drugs

The World Health Organization has defined an ADR as:

> a response to a drug which is noxious and unintended, and which occurs at doses normally used in man for the prophylaxis, diagnosis or therapy of disease or for the modification of a physiological function.
>
> (WHO, 1970)

It is important to always ensure that a risk assessment is completed and a risk management plan is initiated in case a patient has an ADR or a near miss.

The MHRA followed the WHO definition for ADRs as 'noxious and unintended responses to a medicinal product' (WHO, 1969). Elliot et al. (2018) found that approximately 712 deaths per year were because of avoidable ADRs, with an estimate ranging from 1,700 to 22,303 deaths a year. The research concluded that 'Ubiquitous medicines use in health care leads unsurprisingly to high numbers of medication errors, although most are not clinically important'. Of a total estimated 237 million medication errors, researchers found that almost three in four were unlikely to result in harm to patients (Elliot et al., 2018).

Case Study: A Nurse in Pennsylvania Was Fatigued and Forgot to Administer the Second of Two Chemotherapy Treatments to a Patient (lessons to be learnt)

How It Happened
   The nurse had worked a 12-hour shift but decided to stay on longer to help her team. Earlier that day, one of her patients had been diagnosed with cancer, so she was now responsible for administering two doses of their chemotherapy treatment. The nurse put one of the doses in a drawer for safekeeping and administered the other to the patient. Once she finished administering the first dosage, she headed home forgetting about the second dose.
   The next medication dose was administered the following day. No adverse effects were experienced by the patient.

(https://www.berxi.com/resources/articles/medication-errors-in-nursing/)

Thinking Point

Reflect on how this could have possibly happened.
   What measures would you implement to prevent or minimise the likelihood of this.

Patients or clinicians should report suspected adverse drug reactions (ADRs) due to an allergy if:

• The reaction occurred while the patient was being treated with the drug, or
• The drug is known to cause this pattern of reaction, or
• The patient has had a similar reaction to the same drug or drug-class previously.
• A suspected reaction is less likely to be caused by a drug allergy if there is a possible non-drug cause or if there are only gastro-intestinal symptoms present.
                    (Adverse reactions to drugs | Medicines guidance | BNF | NICE)

The principle of pharmacovigilance (above) is also relevant for the reporting of adverse reactions, including those for Black triangle medications. Black triangle drugs are newly licensed, a combination of two older drugs, use of drugs for a different indication in a different patient population as well as a different method of delivery or route. Black triangle drugs are identified by an inverted triangle sign.

The Yellow Card scheme commenced in 1964, following the thalidomide disaster. Initially doctors, dentists and coroners were provided with prep-paid cards for reporting any suspected reactions to licensed drugs. Today pharmacists, nurses and midwives and other prescribing clinicians as well as the patient and carers may report any adverse reactions. ADRs may result from a known effect as well as from a new, hitherto unknown side effect. ADRs must be reported to the MHRA as directed below.

Suspected ADRs should be reported through the Yellow Card Scheme at the following website: http://www.mhra.gov.uk/yellowcard. This should include:

...medicines, vaccines, herbal, homeopathic or complementary products, whether self-medicated or prescribed. This includes suspected adverse drug reactions associated with misuse, overdose, medication errors or from use of unlicensed and off-label medicines. Yellow Cards can also be used to report medical device incidents, defective medicines, and suspected fake medicines. (MHRA, https://bnf.nice.org.uk/medicines-guidance/adverse-reactions-to-drugs/#:~:text=Suspected%20adverse%20drug%20reactions%20should,whether%20self%2Dmedicated%20or%20prescribed)

Matters for reporting on the MHRA's Yellow Card website include defective medicine in terms of quality, fake medicines or faulty medical devices and safety concerns such as those related to e-cigarettes or e-liquids. The aim of reporting is to collect data which may be useful in identifying and managing risks. Healthcare professionals are required by law to report suspected ADRs on the Yellow Card reporting system – this is regardless of whether you prescribed the drug or not. A patient or their carer can report.

Wrongful actions; errors, misdiagnosis, prescriptions and administration

Risk is always present and, far too often, patients may be harmed if there is a lack of or poor risk assessment and management. It is a question of minimising harm to an acceptable level as it is humanly not possible to eliminate it. The six most common areas of risk with medicines across health and adult social care were identified as:

1   Prescribing, monitoring and reviewing
2   Administration
3   Transfer of care
4   Reporting and learning from incidents
5   Supply, storage and disposal
6   Staff competence and workforce capacity
                    (CQC, 2019, https://www.cqc.org.uk/publications/major-report/
                                        medicines-health-social-care)

An action for personal injury due to clinical negligence may be initiated following wrongful actions (see Chapter 2). A patient may be harmed due to a misdiagnosis or a missed opportunity, and the consequence may be detrimental to their health, with resulting avoidable harm. When systemic failures may be suspected, and reported, the HSE or the Care Quality Commission (CQC) may investigate and enforce improvement notices or even prosecute a healthcare provider and their employees subject to sections 2 and 7 of HASAWA (1974). If intent or gross negligence is established, a patient who falls victim to clinical negligence may also recover damages for personal injury under Tort Law. If criminal intent or gross negligence manslaughter is evident, criminal prosecution under section 47 of the Offences against the Person Act 1861 may follow. Healthcare professionals may also be referred to their Professional Regulatory Body with resulting disciplinary action (see Chapter 2).

Case Study

In September 2016, CQC successfully prosecuted a care home provider and a registered manager. Both failed to provide safe care and treatment resulting in avoidable harm.

A 78-year-old man with vascular dementia relied on the provider and registered manager to make sure he received his medicines safely. Two weeks after moving to the service, the man was admitted to hospital and discharged four days later on anticoagulant therapy. He was discharged with an 18-day supply of medicine. The provider and manager failed to order a new prescription after the 18 days. Their systems failed to identify that the medication was missed for between 30 and 33 days.

The man died from a pulmonary thromboembolism and deep vein thrombosis.

CQC's investigation uncovered other unsafe medicines practices for this man, including:

incorrectly transcribing prescriptions, having only one staff member booking medicines in, when two were required, gaps in the administration of medicines, continuing at a higher dose when the dose should have been reduced, poor recording on medicine administration records.

In relation to other people using the service, the following errors in medicines management were identified:

- omissions in prescribed medicines
- medicines frequently out of stock
- failure to record allergies
- failure to record times and dosages of medicines.

The provider was ordered to pay: £50,000 fine, £120 victim surcharge
The registered manager was ordered to pay: £665 fine, £66 victim surcharge

(https://www.cqc.org.uk/guidance-providers/learning-safety-incidents/issue-5-safe-management-medicines)

Thinking Point

What recommendations would you make to prevent a similar incident from
happening again?

Risk assessment and risk management should be part of everyday healthcare
delivery in partnership with the patient and this, '…should be seen as a basic human right. As health care is predominantly a service, it is always co-produced with
the users. Achieving safe care requires that patients be informed, involved, and
treated as full partners in their own care' (WHO, 2023). Patients who are victims
may litigate, seeking damages in compensation for personal injury in Tort (Delict)
Law, see Chapter 4). The UK Central Alerting System (CAS) is responsible for
communicating with pharmacies and healthcare providers, sending national patient
safety alerts (PSAs) regarding:

National patient alerts are issued by the Central Alerting System to communicate actions required by healthcare providers to be undertaken to reduce the
risk of death or disability.

(Specialist Pharmacy Service, 2022, https://www.sps.nhs.
uk/articles/responding-to-medication-safety-alerts-and-
notifications/#:~:text=National%20Patient%20
Safety%20alerts%20are,risk%20of%20
death%20or%20disability)

Conclusion

There is no doubt that medications management is a priority and an essential aspect
of treatment. All clinicians have a duty of care, to be aware of their duty of care
in law to ensure that they minimise the risk, so patients are not harmed. Safety is
achieved by conducting appropriate risk assessments and putting in place risk management plans with appropriate interventions which promote the patient's wellbeing and physical and mental health recovery. This also means that interventions
must be evaluated timely for their effectiveness.

If objectives of treatment are met, this should be to ensure the efficacy or
lack of it. This is to continue monitoring. Considering the requirement for pharmacovigilance (as highlighted earlier), this is essential for patient's safety. It is
also part of professionalism and the ethical and legal duty of care to ensure that
patients are kept safe and not harmed through unsafe practice in treatment and
poor management of medicines and medicinal products. Patient safety comes
first.

References

BNF (2023) available online at;https://bnf.nice.org.uk/ accessed on 23rd October 2023

Care Quality Commission (2017) Available online at: https://www.cqc.org.uk/publications/major-reports/cqc-insight-14-medicines-safety-nhs-trusts

Courtney Griffiths (2010) Independent and supplementary prescribing, an essential guide. Cambridge: Cambridge University Press

CQC (2016) Case study. Available online at: https://www.cqc.org.uk/guidance-providers/learning-safety-incidents/issue-5-safe-management-medicines (Accessed on 22nd May 2024)

CQC (2019) Medicines in health and adult social care: Learning from risks and sharing good practice for better outcomes, CQC-435-062019. Available online at: www.cqc.org.uk

Crown Report (1989). Available online at: https://www.publichealth.hscni.net/directorate-nursing-and-allied-health-professions/nursing/nurse-prescribing (Accessed on 20th November 2023)

Cumberlege Report (1986) Neighbourhood nursing: A focus for care. Available online at: https://www.publichealth.hscni.net/directorate-nursing-and-allied-health-professions/nursing/nurse-prescribing

Cumberlege Report (2020) First do no harm: The report of the independent medicines and medical devices safety review. Available online at: https://www.immdsreview.org.uk/downloads/IMMDSReview_Web.pdf

DoH (2004) Management of medicines, a resource to support implementation of the wider aspects of medicines management for the national service frameworks for diabetes, renal services and long-term conditions. Available online at: http://webarchive.nationalarchives.gov.uk/20121101234412/http://www.dh.gov.uk/prod_consum_dh/groups/dh_digitalassets/@dh/@en/documents/digitalasset/dh_4088755.pdf(Accessed on 20th November 2023)

Donoghue v Stevenson (1932) UKHL 100

Elliot RA, Camacho E, Jankovic D, Sculpher MJ, Faria R (2018) Economic analysis of the prevalence and clinical and economic burden of medication error in England, *BMJ Quality and Safety* 30. Available online at: 10.1136/bmjqs-2019-010206 (Accessed on 20th November 2023)

Health and Safety at Work Act (1974) Sections 2 and 7

Health and Social Care Act (2001) Available online at: https://www.legislation.gov.uk/ukpga/2001/15/contents (Accessed on 23rd May 2024)

Human Medicines Regulations (2012)

Marino M, Jamal Z, Zito P (2023) Pharmacodynamics. National Library of Medicine, PubMed Publishing. Available online at: https://pubmed.ncbi.nlm.nih.gov/29939568/ (Accessed on 22nd May 2024)

Medicinal Products, Prescription by Nurses Act (1992) Available online at: https://www.legislation.gov.uk/ukpga/1992/28 (Accessed on 22nd May 2024)

Medicines Act (1968)

Mental Capacity Act (2005)

Mental Health Act (1983) Sections 2–5

MHRA (2020) Medicinal products definition. Available online at: https://assets.publishing.service.gov.uk/government/uploads/system/uploads/attachment_data/file/872742/GN8_FINAL_10_03_2020__combined_.pdf (Accessed on 20th November 2023)

Misuse of Drugs Act (1971) (as amended 2010)

Misuse of Drugs Regulations (2001)

Misuse of Drugs Regulations (2005)

Montgomery (Appellant) v Lanarkshire Health Board (Respondent) (2015) UKSC 11. Available online at: https://www.oxbridgenotes.co.uk/law_cases/montgomery-v-lanarkshire-health-board#:~:text=The%20ruling%20in%20Montgomery%20v,comprehensive%20information%20to%20their%20patients

Mulac A, Taxis K, Hagesaether E, Granas A (2021) Severe and fatal medication errors in hospitals: Findings from the Norwegian incident reporting system, Eur J Hosp Pharm 2021. Available online at: 10.1136/ejhpharm-2020-002298 (Accessed on 20th November 2023)

National Patients Safety Agency (2007) Safety in doses: Medication safety incidents in the NHS. Available online at: https://www.npsa.gov.uk/ (Accessed on 20th November 2023)

NHS England (2023a) Best practice guidance on safe use of O_2 cylinders. Available online at: http://www.hse.gov.uk/risk/fivesteps.htm (Accessed on 20th November 2023)

NHS England (2023b) Use of oxygen cylinders where patients do not have access to medical gas pipeline systems. Available online at: http://www.hse.gov.uk/risk/fivesteps.htm

NHS Health England (2023) Training for non-medical prescribers. Health Education England. Available online at: https://www.hee.nhs.uk/our-work/medicines-optimisation/training-non-medical-prescribers (Accessed on 20th November 2023)

NHS Plan (2000) 10-year plan. Available online at: https://www.kingsfund.org.uk/publications/nhs-10-year-plan

NICE (2023) Import and safety of controlled drugs. Available online at: https://bnf.nice.org.uk/medicines-guidance/controlled-drugs-and-drug-dependence/ (Accessed on 21st November 2023)

Nursing Notes (2015, 2018). Available online at: https://nursingnotes.co.uk/resources/10-rights-of-medication-administration/ (Accessed on 21st November 2023)

Prendergast v Sam Dee Ltd and Others (1989)

Patient Safety Commissioner Office. Available online at: https://www.patientsafetycommissioner.org.uk/our-work/history/ (Accessed on 21st November 2023)

Royal College of Psychiatrists (2019) How effective is ECT? Available online at: https://www.rcpsych.ac.uk/mental-health/treatments-and-wellbeing/ect (Accessed on 21st November 2023)

Royal Pharmaceutical Society (2013) Medicines optimisation, helping patients to make the most of medicines. Available online at: https://www.rpharms.com/Portals/0/RPS%20document%20library/Open%20access/Policy/helping-patients-make-the-most-of-their-medicines.pdf (Accessed on 23rd November 2023)

Scally G and Donaldson LJ (1998) Clinical governance and the drive for quality improvement in the new NHS in England, BMJ, 317(7150), 61–65

Specialist Pharmacy Service (2022). Available online at: https://www.sps.nhs.uk/ (Accessed on 23rd November 2023)

Thomson A (2009) Back to basics: Pharmacokinetics, PJ, June 2004, 15, 28. Available online at: https://pharmaceutical-journal.com/article/ld/back-to-basics-pharmacokinetics (Accessed on 20th January 2024)

Waller P (2009) An introduction to pharmacovigilance. Oxford: Wiley-Blackwell

WHO (1969) Health organization. International drug monitoring: Technical report series no. 425. [Page 6]. Geneva: World Health Organization

WHO (1970) International drug monitoring: The role of the hospital. WHO Report. Drug Intell Clin Pharm, 4, 101–110.

WHO (2020) Pharmacovigilance. Available online at: https://www.who.int/teams/regulation-prequalification/regulation-andsafety/pharmacovigilance#:~:text=Pharmacovigilance%20is%20the%20science%20and,they%20are%20authorized%20for%20use (Accessed on 23rd November 2023)

WHO (2023) Global patient safety action plan 2021–2030: Towards eliminating avoidable harm in health care. Available online at: https://www.who.int/teams/integrated-health-services/patient-safety/policy/global-patient-safety-action-plan#:~:text=The%20action%20plan%20aims%20to,years%20(2021%E2%80%932030) (Accessed on 23rd May 2024)

6 Care of vulnerable people and safety

Paul Buka

Introduction

Clinicians make treatment decisions on a day-to-day basis which may impact the wellbeing of their patients. Such decisions should, where possible, be made in partnership with the patients respecting the latter's right to choose or decline treatment. If they lack capacity, the decision should be in their (patient's) best interests. This issue falls under the umbrella of 'human rights' which emerged after the Second World War. This UN's Universal Declaration of Human Rights 1948 set out people's basic rights and freedoms in 30 articles which are applicable. Subsequently, the United Kingdom became signatory to the European Convention on Human Rights (ECHR) 1950, with 14 articles that derived from this United Nations International Treaty.

In decision-making within clinical settings, healthcare providers, clinicians, and healthcare staff have a duty of care to ensure the safety of their patients (Section 7, Health and Safety at Work Act, HASAWA, 1974).

> Being vulnerable is defined as in need of special care, support, or protection because of age, disability, risk of abuse or neglect.
> (Public Health England, 2020, https://www.gov.uk/government/
> publications/vulnerabilities-applying-all-our-health/
> vulnerabilities-applying-all-our-health)

Vulnerability applies to 'at risk' populations of service users such as children, older people, and those with physical or mental disabilities who fall within more than one category. Any risk assessment and risk management may present challenges due to varying degrees of needs as well as health inequalities for marginalised groups who may experience discrimination. The prospect of negative discrimination is recognised by the 'nine protected characteristics', defined by the Equality Act (2010). Socio-economic factors, deprivation, and affordability may also account for this, for example, people who cannot afford to pay for prescriptions or who may be experiencing inadequate accommodation. In 2018–2020, males living in the most deprived areas were living 9.7 years fewer than males living in the least deprived areas,

DOI: 10.4324/9781003376934-6

with the gap at 7.9 years for females; both sexes have seen statistically significant increases in the inequality in life expectancy at birth since 2015–2017 (Office of National Statistics [ONS], 2022). This pattern was also reflected in all UK countries.

It is also possible that patients from deprived backgrounds may be more vulnerable to co-morbidities and higher levels of dependence affecting their overall wellbeing, Section 2 of HASAWA 1974 requires a healthcare provider a duty of care to ensure the safety of everyone (especially that of vulnerable people) applicable to healthcare environments/settings. Likewise, under section 7, HASAWA 1974, an employee has also a duty of care to ensure the safety of others (with whom they interact) as well as their own. The welfare of a service user depends on the service provider and skills of any given clinician, who has legal and professional obligations to ensure that those in their care are not harmed by their negligent actions or omissions.

Duty of care applies to record-keeping and due to the fiduciary relationship (patient-clinician, which is based on trust). Clinicians have a degree of 'control' with (literary), the patients' lives in their hands. Crucially, an integral aspect of patient care is accurate record-keeping an effective tool for continuity and effectiveness of care, subject to the General Data Protection Regulation (GDPR) in the Data Protection Act (2018). Access to records or patient-care-related information must be on a need-to-know basis. National guidelines on information were set by the Caldicott Guidelines (1997), which are a framework for all data collected for the provision of health and social care services. This is in respect to patient-identifiable information which the patients would expect to remain private.

Principle 1: Justify the purpose(s) for using confidential information.
Principle 2: Use confidential information only when it is necessary.
Principle 3: Use the minimum necessary confidential information.
Principle 4: Access to confidential information should be on a strict need-to-know basis.
Principle 5: Everyone with access to confidential information should be aware of their responsibilities.
Principle 6: Comply with the law.
Principle 7: The duty to share information for individual care is as important as the duty to protect patient confidentiality.
Principle 8: Inform patients and services users about how their confidential information is used and what choice they have. There should be no surprises.
(Caldicott Guidelines, 1997, https://www.themdu.com/
guidance-and-advice/guides/the-caldicott-principles-
and-guardian-roles-explained)

There is also a common law duty of confidentiality placed on the healthcare professional in order to ensure privacy and non-disclosure except as prescribed by the law. In the event of unauthorised disclosure, the patient is entitled to recover damages in litigation for defamation. This principle was established in the following case.

Case Law: AG v Guardian Newspapers Ltd. (No. 2) [1990]

A retired secret service employee sought to publish his memoirs from Australia. The British government sought to restrain publication there. The defendants sought to report those proceedings, which would involve the publication of the allegations made. The AG sought to restrain those publications.

Held: " A duty of confidence arises when confidential information comes to the knowledge of a person (the confidant) in circumstances where he has notice, or is held to have agreed, that the information is confidential, with the effect that it would be just in all the circumstances that he should be precluded from disclosing the information to others."

There are, however, exceptions when disclosure is permissible under the law, for example, with the patient's consent, or by statutes such as the Public Health (Control of Disease) Act 1984 and NHS (Venereal Disease) Regulations (1974), where required by the court or where a person is about to commit a crime. Another exception is 'in the Public Interest' though this could be debatable and open to challenge.

A safer environment for vulnerable patients

A caring relationship is assumed to be on trust and an unequal balance due to the dependence and vulnerability of the patient. Paternalism was by nature a relationship based on trust, meaning that a clinician may be in a position of controlling, influencing or worse still, harming a vulnerable patient. Unfortunately, there have been cases when trust was eroded, and patients were harmed by clinicians' actions or omissions. Vulnerable people may also be at risk due to human factors. As people are living longer, it means that there will be more vulnerable people in need of care.

Over the 10 years between 2011 and 2021, the population of England increased by 6.5% to an estimated 56,536,000, the highest rate of the four countries of the UK; the estimated population of Northern Ireland increased by 5.0% to 1,905,000, Scotland by 3.4% to 5,480,000, and Wales by 1.4% to an estimated 3,105,000.

(ONS, 2021, https://www.ons.gov.uk/peoplepopulationandcommunity/
populationandmigration/populationestimates/bulletins/
annualmidyearpopulationestimates/latest)

Some older people belong to a vulnerable group due to likely frailties and co-morbidities, '…out of a total of 16.6 million hospital admissions in 2017', 3.5 million (22.2%) were people aged 75 years and over and 41.1% of all days spent in hospital (Public Health England, 2020). One possible factor that may negatively affect the quality of healthcare delivery is limited resources, which do not necessarily match the needs of a growing population. Other vulnerable groups may also be at risk. Organisational failures, such as poor staffing levels or poor training or skill mix, and culture as identified in Mid-Staffordshire (Francis Report, 2013). While most healthcare professionals are dedicated and caring, there were, nevertheless, examples of a few who reportedly let patients down, such as Harold Shipman, Colin Norris, Beverley Allitt, Vitorino Chua, and Lucy Letby, who evidently not only put patients at risk but also actively harmed vulnerable people, including children, whose care they had been entrusted with.

Decision-making, informed consent, and best interests

Decision-making is a central aspect of healthcare and goes on all the time within clinical settings. Consent to treatment should therefore be the basis of the patient's agreement to receive any given treatment. Assessing mental capacity can be challenging as an individual's understanding may fluctuate. One example is people with dementia, who may have a mental capacity which is transient or may be valid for one specific issue while not for another aspect. It is important for clinicians to conduct risk assessments to ensure the safety of all receiving care as well as their own safety. The Health and Safety Executive has drawn national guidelines for all environments where people may engage.

Step 1: Identify the hazards which vulnerable may face in practice and weigh the risk to allow only minimum acceptable levels.

Step 2: Decide who might be harmed and how, put measures in place.

Step 3: Evaluate the risks and decide on precautions, and measure against current policy.

Step 4: Record your findings and implement them, record-keeping should follow the GDC standards.

Step 5: Review your assessment and update as necessary, especially in light of action plans.

(Adapted from HSE, 2006, www.hse.gov.uk/pubns)

The challenge for healthcare staff is to ensure that there is, indeed, a thorough and appropriate risk assessment. There is an ongoing need for periodic intervention reviews or evaluations in order to ensure that they are effective or met.

Scenario: Vulnerable Patients: Best Interests and Raising Concerns

On Ward A, an assessment for mental capacity deemed Mr. Z to be competent, even though he had an underlying diagnosis of dementia on a previous admission. Accordingly, Mr Z was allowed to give consent to marriage and the prospective bride engaged the services of a minister, sanctioning the marriage. Every time she came to visit, it was apparent the patient became agitated. He had no known family members. Sadly, the patient passed away in due course, and it emerged that the new wife inherited the estate – no questions asked.

A few months later, nurse Y in Ward A received a telephone call from nurse X in Ward B (same hospital) who told nurse Y that she had a male patient, who was confused, and had no family. She told her that a lady regularly visited him and professing her love for him and wished to be married. Nurse Y recognised the visiting lady's name, though not entirely sure if this was the same lady. She raised concerns, reported this matter to her line manager, and advised nurse X to get in touch with the patient's Community Psychiaric Nurse, (CPN) or District Nurse (DN) and if he had neither of these to arrange for the appointment of an independent advocate. It turned out to be the same woman as in the first case.

Thinking Point

1 Identify your workplace policy on safeguarding and whistleblowing?
2 How would you have dealt with the situation in the above scenario?

Consent to treatment must be given by a person who has the competence or mental capacity to make a free choice. There must be no deception, duress, incentives, or bribery to influence their choice. For consent to be valid, a patient must be competent to take a relevant decision, have received a sufficient degree of information, and not acting under duress or undue influence (DH, 2009).

There are three elements of validity of properly obtained consent as follows:

- Voluntary – the decision to either consent or not to consent to treatment must be made by the patient themselves and must not be influenced by pressure from clinicians, family, and friends. This means that there should be no incentives offered to the patient or veiled pressures on adverse consequences should they decline treatment, only facts (as it is) should be given.
- Informed – the person must be provided a sufficient degree of information in terms of the nature of the proposed treatment including the benefits and the risks. The clinician should also advise on whether there are reasonable alternatives as well as the detriments or what is likely to happen if the proposed treatment is not followed. They must also discuss alternative treatments as well as what will happen if the proposed treatment doesn't go ahead.
- Capacity is relevant as the person must be capable or has the capacity to give consent. This means that they understand the information provided and that they can use it to make an informed decision.

(NHS Choices, 2016, https://www.nhs.uk/conditions/consent-to-treatment/#:~:text=Consent%20to%20treatment%20means%20a,an%20explanation%20by%20a%20clinician)

Types of consent

Expressed or express is usually described as written or verbal following a 'sufficient degree of understanding' to enable them to make an informed decision. People who are deaf and dumb may also use sign language. There should be evidence (such as words, hand or head signal) that the patient has understood the nature of the treatment, this includes the benefits as well as the potential risks and alternative treatment. They must have clearly expressed their 'agreement, with any proposed treatment'. The mere absence of an objection would not suffice. Written evidence of agreeing, such as a surgical consent form to a proposed treatment or procedure, is more credible in a court of law.

Consent may cover related procedures, provided this is transparent and indicated on the consent form. A patient should never be rushed in decision-making, and they also have a right to change their mind whether they have signed a consent form or not. Verbal consent may be open to challenge should the patient forget.

Explicit Consent (clear) is the basis to explain that a patient outwardly and visibly demonstrates consent. This is like expressed consent and is related to the act of consent given, being clearly evidenced, or witnessed.

Implied Consent – or implicit consent – may also be open to challenge due to the unreliability and interpretation of sign language. This may vary for different people. For example, opening one's mouth may be a sign that a patient accepted consuming oral medication or offering an arm or leg in anticipation of an injection. A clinician must understand the procedure and provide a sufficient degree of information for agreement by the patient. Potential issues can emerge where there are language or cultural barriers.

The patient's best interests should be served if the consent could not be obtained or is unobtainable. In an emergency, two consultants may consent on a patient's behalf. Furthermore, where a service user requires urgent mental health treatment for health issues, they may be sectioned under Sections 2–5, Mental Health Act (MHA, 1983). Best interests override the legal requirement, for example, in an emergency trauma patient. In such cases, two consultants may consent on behalf of a patient lacking capacity.

Case Study: Martha's Rule (2024)

Martha Mills died in 2021 after developing sepsis in a hospital, where she had been admitted with a pancreatic injury after falling off her bike. Martha's family's concerns about her deteriorating condition were not responded to promptly, and in 2023, a coroner ruled that Martha would probably have survived had she been moved to intensive care earlier.

(https://www.england.nhs.uk/patient-safety/marthas-rule/)

New changes for supporting patient's 'best interests' will be introduced by the Martha's rule from April 2024. This meaning that patients, loved ones, and families will have a 'round the clock access to a rapid review from a separate care team if there are concerns about a patient's condition'.

If consent is knowingly or unknowingly improperly superseded by a healthcare professional, a patient may raise an action for a breach of human rights against a public body employing any healthcare professional in question. Healthcare employees should report this.

Article 1: Everyone's right to life shall be protected by law.
Article 3: Prohibition of torture and,
Article 8: Right to respect for private and family life.
1 Everyone has the right to respect for his private and family life, his home, and his correspondence.
No one shall be subjected to torture or to inhuman or degrading treatment or punishment.

(European Convention on Human Rights [ECHR], 1950; Human Rights Act, 1998)

The principle of the right to refuse treatment is illustrated by the principle established in a well-known US case (below), which is defined as *(persuasive and not a precedent in UK law)* which is related to individual autonomy and the right to refuse treatment, are found in the summary below:

Case Law: Schloendorff v. Society of New York Hospital, 211 NY, 105 NE 92, 93 (1914)

This was a case where a woman had consented to an abdominal examination, under anaesthesia but not to a surgical operation. Knowing this to be the case the surgeon went ahead to operate and remove a tumour. The patient successfully sued for battery.

Held, Justice Cardozo's opinion (at p. 304) expressed what has now become the foundation for the concept of informed consent and for an individual patient's right to autonomy and self-determination.

Every human being of adult years and sound mind has a right to determine what shall be done with his own body; and a surgeon who performs an operation without his patient's consent commits an assault for which he is liable in damages.

(Schloendorff v. Society of New York Hospital, 211 NY, 105 NE 92, 93 (1914), 106 N.E. 93 (N.Y. 1914))

Thinking Point

1 The above is an American case, which is often cited but not necessarily followed as a precedent and not binding in the United Kingdom and across Common Law jurisdictions.
2 Consider what should happen in respect of consent in emergency situations.

Subject to Criminal Law, a person who fails to obtain informed consent may be charged with battery (or assault in Scotland), subject to the Offences Against the Person Act 1861, Section 42 for common assault, and Section 47 for inflicting actual bodily harm. A person committing common assault or battery may be imprisoned or required to pay fines plus costs (see Chapter 4).

Patients have a right to refuse treatment if, on admission to a hospital, have a "Living Will," and this may in fact be either an Advance Decision or an Advance Statement. These would only be valid if the person who made them had mental capacity at the time they were made. All staff should be made aware.

Advance Statement – This is NOT legally binding but must be used to inform care-planning.

An example is the indication of a preferred place of care document which states that a person would prefer to initiate or continue with palliative treatment and supported to die at home.

Advance Decision – Legally binding and must be followed.

On example is a written statement from a person's solicitor which states they do not wish to be resuscitated in the event of cardio-respiratory arrest. Clinicians must always ask to see written proof of an advanced directive and escalate to clarify its validity. Under Section 24 (1) of the Mental Capacity Act (MCA) 2005 Adults with Incapacity (Scotland) Act 2000, a person may make Advance Decisions to refuse treatment: generally, assuming he is at least 18 years old and has the capacity at the time to make an Advance Directive (confer on Chapter 7).

Consent for children (under the age of 16) and safety

The World Health Organisation (WHO, 2023) has a wide definition of adolescents as, "… individuals in the 10-19 years age group and 'youth' as the 15–24-year age group. While 'Young People' covers the age range 10–24 years".

In the United Kingdom, however, subject to s 11, Children Act (2004), the safeguarding duty of care for vulnerable children falls upon local authorities. Nevertheless, children aged between 10 and 17 themselves are subject to the age of criminal responsibility under the Children and Young Persons Act (1963). Should they commit a crime, children within this age range can be arrested and taken to court. However, they will be tried in youth Courts and if found guilty, when it comes to sentencing, they are dealt with differently with somewhat lighter terms and committed to special secure centres for young people but not to adult prisons. Children aged 16 can legally consent to sexual activity, join the army, and they can also drive. From the age or 17 or 16 they can legally have sex with anyone else above this age. It is however illegal to sext anyone under the age of 18.

When it comes to treatment, any person aged 16 and over is deemed competent to give consent to treatment. There is, however, a presumption in law that a child below 16 is 'incompetent', and a person with parental responsibility must consent on that child's behalf. Parental responsibilities are of duties and not 'rights' over their child's. On competence for those below the age of 16, healthcare professionals are guided by the Gillick case that established the Gillick Competence. This is also defined as the so-called Fraser Guidelines in the following case:

Case Law: Gillick v West Norfolk and Wisbech HA [1986]

- A DHSS circular stated that in certain circumstances, a doctor could lawfully prescribe contraception for a girl under 16 without the consent of the parents.
- Mrs Gillick challenged this in the courts, arguing that children below the age of 16 were *not* competent to consent on their own behalf and that the circular adversely affected her ability to discharge her duties as a parent.
- *Held*: "…The principle is that parental right or power of control of the person and property of his child exists primarily to enable the parent to discharge his duty of maintenance, protection and education until he reaches such an age as to be able to look after himself and make his own decisions'…" per Lord Scarman.

The above legal principle (Gillick Case) means that there is no longer age limit. The Gillick Competence, otherwise called Fraser Guidelines, is applicable. This is open to challenge. It is a question of assessing their (child's) intelligence, competence, and understanding of the treatment and implications of informed consent. The court's view was that children of an age lower than 16 may agree to treatment without parental consent or knowledge. Questions may arise if a young person (below the age of 16) does not wish to involve or inform their parents about 'treatment' decisions, for example, prescribing contraceptives.

Persons with mental health needs and mental capacity

The definition of Mental Health is,

"… any disorder or disability of the mind…", - not included are '…those with: - a history of substance misuse and those with Learning Disabilities, (unless associated with 'abnormally aggressive or seriously irresponsible conduct on his part').

(MHA, 1983, (section 1 [2]), as amended by the MHA, 2007)

Individual freedom is a fundamental human right linked to consent to treatment which is under Articles 3, 5, and 8 of the Human Rights Act 1998 (ECHR, 1950) unless a person lacks capacity.

Examples of exceptions of lawful detention are DoLS, MHA (1983). Incarceration in police cells or prison is subject to the provisions of the law.

There may nevertheless be circumstances in which a person with mental health illness may require (in their best interest) compulsory detention and sectioning for treatment under Sections 2–5 of MHA 1983. This means that the service user may be detained and have medication administered without their expressed consent. However, this does not mean that they lose their right to make an informed choice.

Furthermore, subject to Section 135 of the MHA 1983 – if a person is a threat, or at risk to themselves or others, police are empowered to remove a person from his or her home, and this must be done under a warrant from a Justice of the Peace. Furthermore, Section 136 of the same statute also empowers police to remove individual from public place (as an emergency necessity) to a 'place of safety', and they may be subject to detention under Section 5(2) of the MHA for up to 72 hours.

The fact that a person has a diagnosis of mental illness should not justify a presumption that they lack mental capacity. The same test for assessing capacity should be applied. This was clearly the case in Re C below.

Case Law: Re C: (Adult: Refusal of Medical Treatment): 1994(1) All ER

C. was an adult detained in Broadmoor psychiatric hospital.

He had gangrene in his left leg and doctors considered that amputation was necessary to save his life. He refused such treatment.

Although he had a confirmed diagnosis of paranoid schizophrenia, this did not preclude him as automatically incapable of deciding about his medical treatment. The courts considered that he passed the three-stage test and therefore deemed to have capacity to give or withhold the proposed treatment.

Held on appeal that he had mental capacity to make a choice.

Lord Thorpe, re C three-stage test

- Understand in simple language what the medical treatment is, its purpose and nature, and why it is being proposed.
- Understand its principal benefits, risks, and alternatives.
- Understand in broad terms what will be the consequences of not receiving the proposed treatment.

Should a mental capacity test indicate absence of capacity to make decisions, the 'best interests' principle is applied (confer on next section). This means that the Court of Protection may appoint a deputy to advocate for a person who lacks capacity, or they (the patient) may themselves have appointed another individual (while they had their capacity to do so), as their Power of Attorney.

Mental capacity, best interests, and deprivation of liberty safeguards (DoLS [to LPS])

The NHS Constitution (2012) required service user involvement in decision-making about their own treatment and care, and the service user has a right to make decisions related to their own treatment.

Freedom from incarceration is a fundamental rights. Unwarranted holding of a person could be in breach of the Human rights under Article 5 of the ECHR (1950). This defines a person's right *not* to be detained against their wishes, Section 1 of the MCA (2005), was brought in directly to authorise in their best interests. Such was the case in *R v Bournewood Community and Mental Health NHS Trust ex part L. HL 1998 (HL v UK 45508/99 [2004] ECHR 471)* was a case of a man with severe autism and challenging behaviour. It was argued that detention of a man with autism could be justified under the common law doctrine of necessity. However, on appeal to the European Court of Human Rights, it was ruled that R should not be detained unless this was under the MHA. Detention was in contravention of Article 5 of the (ECHR) Human Rights Act 1998 Article 5 (1) and (4) Right to Liberty and Security (imprisonment). This case triggered the introduction of the DoLS (in 2009) in the MCA (2005), and this means that holding a person in detention may be lawful if they lack capacity. The justification would be that, such an action is in their best interests, as provided for by statute. DoLS MCA (2005) is applicable, in their best interests, i.e., for their own safety. DoLS at the time of writing is due to be replaced by Liberty Protection Safeguards (LPS) – implementation possibly in late-2024 or beyond.

Section 4 of the MCA (2005) provides a checklist.

These five principles are the following:

1 Presumption of capacity.
2 Support to decide.
3 Ability to make unwise decisions.
4 Best interest.
5 Least restrictive.

(Brain Injury Group, https://www.braininjurygroup.
co.uk/news/principles-mental-capacity-act/)

The fourth and fifth principles apply only when a person has been assessed to not have mental capacity for the decision in question. A patient may lack capacity in one aspect and yet have a sufficient degree of understand in another, hence it is important, as required by statute, that patients are assessed for all decisions relating to specific treatment.

The MCA (2005) considers limitations such as communication and sensory deficit. Under Section 37 of the same act, the court may make an order to place a person who lacks capacity to hospital instead of prison. There is need for separation of a lack of incapacity and mental health illness. The leading case is the *Cheshire West*, it illustrates this point below. For DoLS to be lawful in order to allow lawfully depriving a person of their freedom, they must be over the age of 18 (under the anticipated LPS, the age minimum has been lowered to over 16) and the person may be residing in their own home. Deprivation of liberty must be in their best interests, with family consent, and necessary for their welfare.

Case Law: P v Cheshire West and Chester Council and another and P and Q v Surrey County Council [2014] UKSC 19, [2014] MHLO 16

This involved a 38-year-old man with Cerebral Palsy & Down's syndrome, living in bungalow with two other residents supervised by two staff during the day and one at night. He was able to attend a day centre, pool pub, and club with constant supervision due to incontinence and constantly pulling off his incontinence nappies.

The Supreme Court judgement

The ACID TEST:

This is applied in deciding whether an incapacitated adult is being deprived of their liberty which comprises two key questions:

A person is deprived of his liberty if he

1   Is the person subject to (a) continuous **supervision** and, (b) **control**? and
2   Is the person {c] **free to leave**?
    If this is the case, being then they are derived of their liberty.

(http://supremecourt.uk/decided-cases/docs/UKSC_2012_0068_Judgment.pdf)

Current provisions are applicable to persons who are resident in hospitals or residential care and lack capacity to decide. On application, the Court of Protection may appoint a suitable person to be a 'litigation friend' to represent a person who lacks capacity in the Court of Protection, for example, and they are:

• a parent or guardian;
• a family member or friend;
• a solicitor;

- a professional advocate, for example, an Independent Mental Capacity Advocate (IMCA) ;
- a Court of Protection deputy; and
- someone who has a lasting or enduring power of attorney.

(https://www.gov.uk/litigation-friend/suitability)

If there is no person available or willing to take on the role of a 'litigation friend,' the court may appoint a legally qualified 'Official Solicitor' to represent a person who lacks capacity. Vulnerable people were provided for by the Social Care Act (2014), requiring a general duty on Local Authorities to conduct a needs assessment for persons living in the community who need care.

Client abuse and safeguarding

Vulnerable persons may fall victim to abuse at the hands of a trusted individual such as healthcare professionals, carers, and family members. Client abuse is defined as

> ... any behaviour towards a service user that is an offence under the Sexual Offences Act (2003)(a), ill-treatment (whether of a physical or psychological nature) of a service user, theft, misuse or misappropriation of money or property belonging to a service user, or. neglect of a service user.

(CQC, Regulation 13, 2023)

There are several classifications of abuse affecting vulnerable people such as older people, children, and people with disabilities, current categories of abuse include the following:

- Physical abuse
- Domestic violence or abuse
- Sexual abuse
- Psychological or emotional abuse
- Financial or material abuse
- Modern slavery
- Discriminatory abuse
- Organisational or institutional abuse
- Neglect or acts of omission
- Self-neglect

(Social Care Institute for Excellence, https://www.scie.org.uk/safeguarding/adults/introduction/types-and-indicators-of-abuse)

The term 'abuse' applies to any settings including hospitals and communities as well as domestic ones. Since 2021, however, there has been a shift towards a focus recognising abuse within domestic settings. There will be similarities between types of abuse which is found in institutions such as residential care-homes, nursing homes, and domestic environments. Detecting domestic abuse can be more of a challenge for healthcare professionals due to often hidden signs of abuse in the community. This is because when clinicians ask questions on admission assessments of 'risk', vulnerable service users may protect an abuser or not wish to cooperate or necessarily show obvious signs of abuse. The most recent definition of abuse also now focuses on the domestic aspect, extending the concept, thus making it more of a challenge to detect potential abuse.

The Domestic Abuse Act (2021) and the Domestic Abuse (Protection) (Scotland) Act 2021 widened the categories, with a comprehensive definition of domestic abuse:

1   This section defines "domestic abuse" for the purposes of this Act.
2   Behaviour of a person ("A") towards another person ("B") is "domestic abuse" if –

   a   A and B are each aged 16 or over and are personally connected to each other, and
   b   the behaviour is abusive.

3   Behaviour is "abusive" if it consists of any of the following:

   a   Physical or sexual abuse.
   b   Violent or threatening behaviour.
   c   Controlling or coercive behaviour.
   d   Economic abuse (see subsection (4)).
   e   Psychological, emotional, or other abuse; and it does not matter whether the behaviour consists of a single incident or a course of conduct.
                    (https://www.legislation.gov.uk/ukpga/2021/17/section/1/enacted)

What the above statute aims to achieve is to extend the statutory definition of abuse from not only physical aspects but also to emotional and controlling, coercive behaviour, and economic abuse. Assessment of a victim with signs of suspected abuse can be challenging for a clinician. It may be a challenge for healthcare professionals undertaking a physical and/or a psychological examination. A potential victim of abuse may refuse to cooperate for fear of retribution from an alleged abuser or the impact of the abuser being punished and/or removed for their own safety under the Care Act 2014 and Care (Scotland) Act 2014. The causes of abuse may be varied depending on individual circumstances. Unfortunately, a significant number of victims may experience abuse at the hands of a partner. Healthcare staff must report any signs of abuse (even if it turns out that they were wrong, rather than do nothing). Victims may be in denial and present with anxiety, post-traumatic disorder, depression, or substance and/or alcohol abuse (El Serag and Thurston, 2020). The classification of specifically domestic abuse was captured by the ONS international figures as follows, with figures rising by 9% in 2020. For the 12-month period to the year ending March 2020:

> ...the Crime Survey for England and Wales showed that an estimated 2.3 million adults aged 16 to 74 years experienced domestic abuse in the last year (1.6 million women and 757,000 men), a slight but non-significant decrease from the previous year. The police recorded 758,941 domestic abuse-related crimes in England and Wales.
>
> (ONS, 2020, https://www.ons.gov.uk/peoplepopulationandcommunity/ crimeandjustice/bulletins/domesticabuseinenglandandwalesoverview/ november2020)

Service users receiving physical and/or psychological care require a comprehensive risk assessment and risk management plan that is holistic. Shared decision-making requires consent and concordance in the treatment plan. This should also empower the service user and ensure that the risk of potential harm is fully assessed, identified, and minimised, if not removable.

On reporting abuse, Section 42 of the Social Care Act (2014) requires an investigation by the responsible local authority.

1 This section applies where a local authority has reasonable cause to suspect that an adult in its area (whether ordinarily resident there) –

   a has needs for care and support (whether or not the authority is meeting any of those needs),
   b is experiencing, or is at risk of, abuse or neglect, and
   c as a result of those needs is unable to protect himself or herself against the abuse or neglect or the risk of it.

2 The local authority must make (or cause to be made) whatever enquiries it thinks necessary to enable it to decide whether any action should be taken in the adult's case (whether under this Part or otherwise) and, if so, what and by whom.

3 "Abuse" includes financial abuse; and for that purpose, "financial abuse" includes –

   a having money or other property stolen,
   b being defrauded,
   c being put under pressure in relation to money or other property, and
   d having money or other property misused.

> (Section 42 of the Social Care Act, 2014, https://www.legislation. gov.uk/ukpga/2014/23/section/42/enacted)

As part of safeguarding the employer has a duty of care to undertake regular Disclosure and Baring (DBS) checks on staff, usually every three years, safeguarding also includes whistleblowing locally and reporting any concerns to the police as well as the Care Quality Commission (CQC), the Parliamentary and Health Ombudsman for complaints and reporting abuse and also children's commissioner. Following the Cumberlege Report, which was led by Baroness Cumberlege (2020), there was a recommendation for a Patient Safety Commissioner. The main objectives of the Patient Safety Commissioner were the following:

- The independent commissioner will act as a champion for patients and lead a drive to improve the safety of medicines and medical devices,
    and
- … will improve how the healthcare system listens to patients, the government and the NHS to put patients first.

(Department of Health and Social Care, 2022, https://www.
gov.uk/government/news/first-ever-patient-
safety-commissioner-appointed)

The Health and Care Act (2022) introduced legislative measures aiming at a patient-centred approach and for health and care organisations to deliver joined-up care for people who rely on multiple different services. This followed recommendations by NHS England and NHS Improvement.

Its aim was '… to establish a legislative framework that supports collaboration and partnership-working to integrate services for patients. Among a wide range of other measures, the Act also includes targeted changes to public health, social care and the oversight of quality and safety'.

Kings Funds (2022) Act promotes coordination at local levels and dignity and respect, compassion, inclusiveness, and wellbeing. An earlier related statute, Social Care (Self-directed Support) (Scotland) Act 2013 had also taken the patient-centred approach.

Conclusion

Recent positive acknowledgement of the 75th anniversary of the NHS founding also serves as a reminder of where the NHS is and health inequalities, which may put some patients at risk. Some patients from marginalised groups, identified by 'protected characteristics' of the Equality Act (2010), may be more vulnerable, with higher risk of harm in comparison to the wider population. A patient-centred approach to care delivery should enhance decision-making and improved safety. There is now, more than ever, a need for 'joined-up' care, hopefully ensuring that healthcare professionals, social services, and carers are collaborating under the Health and Care Act (2022). This aims to change the focus to patient-centred care and should advance decision-making to improve patient safety.

While acknowledging vulnerability of service users, especially for those with complex needs, it is important for clinicians, carer-givers, or family members to involve and empower patients. Patient-centred care means that vulnerable patients should be supported in decision-making. Only through working in partnership, with advocacy and safeguarding of vulnerable patients, can healthcare staff improve the quality of care and keep them safe.

References

AG v Guardian Newspapers Ltd. (No. 2) [1990] Available online at: https://vlex.co.uk/vid/attorney-general-v-guardian-793420901 (Accessed on 25th May 2014)

Baroness Cumberlege Report – First Do No Harm (2020) The report of the Independent Medicines and Medical Devices Safety Review (IMMDs) Available online at: https://www.hqip.org.uk/the-baroness-cumberlege-report-first-do-no-harm-published-8th-july-2020/ (Accessed on 25th May 2024)

Caldicott Guidelines (1997) Available online at: https://www.themdu.com/guidance-and-advice/guides/the-caldicott-principles-and-guardian-roles-explained (Accessed on 23rd January 2024)

Children Act (1989, 2004)

Children and Young Persons Act (1963) Available online at: https://www.legislation.gov.uk/ukpga/1963/37 (Accessed on 26th May 2024)

CQC (2023) Regulation 13: Safeguarding service users from abuse and improper treatment. Available online at: https://www.cqc.org.uk/guidance-providers/regulations-enforcement/regulation-13-safeguarding-service-users-abuseimproper#:~:text='abuse'%20means%E2%80%94,neglect%20of%20a%20service%20user (Accessed on 2nd December 2023)

Data Protection Act (2018) Available online at: https://www.legislation.gov.uk/ukpga/2018/12/contents

Department of Health (2009) Reference guide to consent for examination or treatment. Available online at: https://assets.publishing.service.gov.uk/government/uploads/system/uploads/attachment_data/file/138296/dh_103653__1_.pdf (Accessed on 3rd November, 2023)

Department of Health and Social Care (2022) Available online at: https://www.gov.uk/government/news/first-ever-patient-safety-commissioner-appointed (Accessed on 25th May 2024)

Domestic Abuse Act (2021) Available online at: https://greenworld.org.uk/article/evaluating-domestic-abuse-act (Accessed on 28th May 2024)

El Serag R, Thurston RC (2020) Matters of the heart and mind: Interpersonal violence and cardiovascular disease in women, Journal of the American Heart Association, 9, e015479. Available online at: https://www.ahajournals.org/doi/full/10.1161/JAHA.120.015479 (Accessed on 24th May 2024)

Equality Act (2010) Available online at: https://www.legislation.gov.uk/ukpga/2010/15/contents (Accessed on 25th May 2024)

European Convention on Human Rights (1950) Available online at: https://www.echr.coe.int/ (Accessed on 23rd December 2023)

Francis Report – Mid Staffordshire (2013) Available online at: https://www.nuffieldtrust.org.uk/research/the-francis-report-one-year-on?gclid=Cj0KCQjwholBhC_ARIsAMpgMoensQD1nT_wLoBWjSUHLpnq68Nh4vCRtQ7hl1skVOTdOGHQw2gGd7waAvOMEALw_wcB (Accessed on 22nd December 2020)

Gillick v West Norfolk & Wisbech AC 112. Health and Social Care Act 2020, available online at: https://www.legislation.gov.uk/ukpga/2022/31/contents accasses on 20th June 2024

Health and Safety at Work Act (1974) Available online at: https://www.hse.gov.uk/legislation/hswa.htm (Accessed on 21st December 2023).

HSE (2006) Available online at: www.hse.gov.uk/pubns (Accessed on 2nd November 2023).

Human Rights Act (1998) Available online at; https://www.legislation.gov.uk/ukpga/1998/42/contents (Accessed on 25th May 2024

Kings Funds (2022) Available online at: https://www.kingsfund.org.uk/publications/health-and-care-act-key-questions (Accessed on 20th December 2023)

Martha's Rule (2024) Available online at: https://www.england.nhs.uk/patient-safety/marthas-rule/ (Accessed on 22th February 2024)

Mental Capacity Act (2005) Available online at: https://www.legislation.gov.uk/ukpga/2005/9/contents (Accessed on 25th May 2024)

Mental Health Act (1983) Available at: https://www.legislation.gov.uk/ukpga/1983/20/contents (Accessed on 25th May 2023)

Mental Health Act (2007) ss2-5, 135, 136 Available online at: https://www.legislation.gov.uk/ukpga/2007/12/contents accessed on 20th June 2024

NHS Choices (2016) Available online at: https://www.nhs.uk/conditions/consent-to-treatment/#:~:text=Consent%20to%20treatment%20means%20a,an%20explanation%20by%20a%20clinician (Accessed on 2nd November 2023)

NHS Constitution (2012) updated 2023. Available online at: https://www.gov.uk/government/publications/the-nhs-constitution-for-england (Accessed on 25th May 2024)

Office of National Statistics (2020) Available online at: https://www.ons.gov.uk/peoplepopulationandcommunity/crimeandjustice/bulletins/domesticabuseinengland andwalesoverview/november2020 (Accessed on 2nd November 2023)

Office of National Statistics (2021) Available online at: https://www.ons.gov.uk/peoplepopulationandcommunity/populationandmigration/populationestimates/bulletins/annualmidyearpopulationestimates/latest

Office of National Statistics (2022) Health inequalities, Health state life expectancies by national deprivation deciles, England: 2018 to 2020. Available online at: https://www.ons.gov.uk/peoplepopulationandcommunity/healthandsocialcare/healthinequalities/bulletins/healthsta telifeexpectanciesbyindexofmultipledeprivationimd/2018to2020 (Accessed on 24th May 2024)

P v Cheshire West and Chester Council and another and P and Q v Surrey County Council (2014) UKSC 19, [2014] MHLO 16

Public Health (Control of Disease) Act (1984) Available online at: https://www.legislation.gov.uk/ukpga/1984/22/contents (Accessed on 25th May 2024)

Public Health England (2020) Older people's hospital admissions in the last year of life. Available online at: https://www.gov.uk/government/publications/older-peoples-hospital-admissions-in-the-last-year-of-life/older-peoples-hospital-admissions-in-the-last-year-of-life#:~:text=There%20were%20a%20total%20of,of%20people%20of%20any%20age (Accessed on 2nd November 2023)

R v Bournewood Community and Mental Health NHS Trust ex part L. HL 1998 (HL v UK 45508/99 [2004] ECHR 471)

Re C: (Adult: Refusal of Medical Treatment): 1994(1) All ER

S 2 Health and Safety at Work Act (1974) Available online at: https://www.hse.gov.uk/legislation/hswa.htm (Accessed on 2nd November 2023).

Schloendorff v. Society of New York Hospital, 211 NY, 105 NE 92, 93 (1914)

Sexual Offences Act (2003) Available online at: https://www.legislation.gov.uk/ukpga/2003/42/contents (Accessed on 23rd May 2024)

Social Care Act (2014) Available online at: https://www.legislation.gov.uk/ukpga/2014/23/contentsavailable (Accessed on 24th May 2024)

Social Care Institute for Excellence. Available online at: https://www.scie.org.uk/safeguarding/adults/introduction/types-and-indicators-of-abuse (Accessed on 2nd November 2023)

Universal Declaration of Human Rights (UN) (1948) Available online at: https://unfoundation.org/what-we-do/issues/peace-human-rights-and-humanitarian-response/?gclid=Cj0KCQjwho-lBhC_ARIsAMpgMoeoUvHeCwziyHWGyPfLSb_9DZKzoEMLZaxn83ZdKRO9cxgTX Keo-CoaAni2EALw_wcB (Accessed on 2nd November 2023)

Venereal Disease Regulation (1974) Available online at: https://www.legislation.gov.uk/uksi/1974/29/made (Accessed on 25th May 2024)

WHO (2023) Adolescent health. Available online at: https://www.who.int/southeastasia/health-topics/adolescent-health#:~:text=WHO%20defines%20%27Adolescents%27%20as%20individuals,15%2D24%20year%20age%20group (Accessed on 2nd November 2023)

7 Leadership, organisational culture and patient safety

David Atkinson and Paul Buka

Introduction

The aim of this chapter is to raise awareness of the impact of leadership on organisations and patient safety and will consider leadership and management styles, along with the duties and responsibilities subject to the Health and Safety at Work Act (HASAWA) 1974. There are numerous publications on theories of leadership and leadership styles, and it is not the purpose or intention of this chapter to regurgitate the plethora of information on these topics but to refer to them when discussing the impact (or the absence) of leadership regarding patient safety. However, it may be useful to start with one of several 'thinking points', and examples included in this chapter, and question some theories about leadership, which Bennis and Nanus (2012) identified as myths.

Thinking Point

Leadership is a rare skill.
  Leaders are born, not made.
  Leaders are charismatic.
  Leadership exists only at the top of an organisation.
  The leader controls, directs, prods, and manipulates.
  Do you agree or disagree with any part or all of the above or do you agree they are myths? If so, why?

Leadership or management

Are leadership and management the same? Not according to Leech (2019), as he suggests that "Management is focused on implementing, organising, measuring, and ensuring everyone is clear on their role and contribution toward the task or goal". This is not quite the same as the role of leadership, which is more abstract and focuses on developing and communicating a vision for the future that

DOI: 10.4324/9781003376934-7

is different to the status quo. Leadership is about encouraging and empowering people to take risks and to innovate (Leech, 2019). For example, consider the duties and responsibilities of leaders in healthcare settings and, in particular, the need to ensure staff adhere to their professional and legal duties, such as in the Health and Safety at Work Act (HASAWA) (Health and Safety Executive, 1974). The HASAWA 1974 – Section 2(1) states that "the employer has a duty to conduct his undertaking in such a way as to ensure, so far as is reasonably practicable, that persons not in his employment who may be affected by the conduct of his undertaking are not as a result exposed to risks to their health and safety". In summary, the main responsibilities are to:

- Provide a safe system of work;
- Provide a safe place of work;
- Provide safe equipment, plant, and machinery; and
- Have safe and competent people working alongside you. Employers are also liable for the actions of their staff and managers.

(Health and Safety Department, 2022)

Are these employers, as leaders, acting purely as managers, or is there any leadership involved, and does it matter either way? Barr and Dowding (2022, p. 16) state that "you do not have to be a manager to be a leader, but you do need to be a good leader to be an effective manager". They go on to suggest a number of differences between leadership and management, though the key differences are that managers are assigned the formally designated role and have authority and influence, whereas leaders have an informal role that is achieved and which involves independent thinking, initiative, and sharing, and most important to note "is part of every healthcare professional's responsibility" (Barr & Dowding, 2022, p. 16).

In addition, if, as the Royal College of Nursing suggested, "everyone is a leader for quality in healthcare" (RCN, 2024), then it is every healthcare professional's responsibility to be accountable as a leader in terms of patient safety. An appropriate definition is "the capacity to influence people, by means of personal attributes and/or behaviours, to achieve a common goal." The question posed is, how is this responsibility and accountability implemented and measured? Where does it start? Government officials are appointed so it would seem they act as managers rather than leaders, and their roles are task orientated and centred on policy making, and they are "a person responsible for managing an organization" (Cambridge Dictionary, no date). This supports the statement, "A manager's primary responsibility is to plan, organise, and control resources to achieve specific goals within an organisation. They focus on managing people, processes, and systems to ensure that operations run smoothly and efficiently" (Flint, 2023). Further to this, do government ministers and policies help or hinder leaders in healthcare by constantly changing legislation and targets and implementing unattainable objectives? According to Kline (2019), the Health and Social Care Act (2012) changed the relationship between Ministers and Arm's Length Bodies, though it had little effect on the way the

NHS workforce was managed and led with, continuing streams of "expectations, requirements, targets, inspections and funding decisions all which fundamentally influence workforce culture and leadership". It was this sequence of events that led Francis (2013) to blame the failings of the Mid Staffordshire Foundation Trust on such a culture that put "the business of the system ahead of patients" and that this culture was more about fear and compliance. The top-down management, exacerbated by government policies, contributed to widespread poor leadership and as a result poor treatment of staff, which in turn led to poor practice and a serious deterioration of the safety and quality of care that patients experienced, occasionally resulting in the death of some of them.

Kline goes on to say that 24% of NHS staff in an England report bullying, harassment, or abuse by fellow workers and managers, leading, amongst other things, to increased intentions to leave and the effectiveness of teams. Evesson and Oxenbridge (2015) state that 'policies, procedures and training' have been viewed as key to "safe, effective means whereby individual staff can raise concerns about bullying, discrimination, unfair disciplinary action and unsafe practice". However, research suggest that this 'methodological individualism' approach is fundamentally flawed as UK employment law is underpinned by its individualistic nature and dominates the treatment of NHS staff. When such an individualistic approach is used, it may also treat toxic leadership as the exception whereas data suggest it is widespread as noted by Aasland et al. (2009).

DePree (2004, p. 1) stated that "Leadership is an Art" in his book of the same name, and Florence Nightingale once said that "Nursing is an Art", though Daft (2017, p. 27) reminds us that leadership is both an art and a science: an art as many of the leadership skills and qualities required cannot be learned, and a science because there is a growing body of knowledge that describes the leadership process. These theories demonstrate how a variety of skills can be used to attain the best and safest possible care for patients. Amongst these skills are the ability to recognise individual strengths of members of a team and to utilise them appropriately, encouraging others to work with their strengths and cultivate latent talents and ensuring that all members of the team communicate effectively.

Team roles and communication

Arguably, the most famous researcher on 'team roles' was Belbin, who came up with the theory that there are nine roles within a team: Shaper, Implementer, Complete-Finisher, Coordinator, Team Worker, Resource Investigator, Plant, Monitor-Evaluator, and Specialist (Belbin, 1981). Belbin's team roles theory comprises different roles within a team, leading to optimal performance. Teams with diverse, complementary roles create innovative solutions and maintain high performance. Clear expectations, communication, and coordination become easier with balanced team roles. One key elements of any role is the effective communication. If this is done appropriately will result in positive outcomes. However, if carried out below standard, the result may be poor practice and performance. The outcome could adversely affect a patient's welfare resulting in a patient's injury or loss of life.

However, when things go wrong, there are the inevitable 'human factors' to take into consideration.

A comprehensive application of Swiss Cheese Model has been analysed by Weigmann et al. (2023)

Organisational Influence

Organisational Culture: Shared values, beliefs, and priorities regarding safety that govern organisational decision-making, as well as the willingness of an organisation to openly communicate and learn from adverse events.

Operational Process: How an organisation plans to accomplish its mission as reflected by its strategic planning, policies/procedures, and corporate oversight.

Resource Management: Support provided by senior leadership to accomplish the objectives of the organisation, including the allocation of human, equipment/facility, and monetary resources.

Supervisory Factors

Inadequate Supervision: Oversight and management of personnel and resources, including training, professional guidance, and engagement.

Planned Inappropriate Operations: Management and assignment of work, including aspects of risk management, staff assignment, work tempo, scheduling, etc.

Failed to Correct Known Problem: Instances in which deficiencies amongst individuals or teams, problems with equipment, or hazards in the environment are known to the supervisor yet are allowed to continue unabated.

Supervisory Violations: The wilful disregard for existing rules, regulations, instructions, or standard operating procedures by managers or supervisors during their duties.

Environmental Factors

Tools and Technology: This category encompasses a variety of issues, including the design of equipment and controls, display/interface characteristics, checklist layouts, task factors, and automation.

Physical Environment: This category includes the setting in which individuals perform their work and consists of such things as lighting, layout, noise, clutter, and workplace design.

Task: Refers to the nature of the activities performed by individuals and teams, such as the complexity, criticality, and consistency of assigned work.

Individual Factors

Mental State: Cognitive/emotional conditions that negatively affect performance such as mental workload, confusion, distraction, memory lapses, pernicious attitudes, misplaced motivation, stress, and frustration.

Physiological State: Medical and/or physiological conditions that preclude safe performance, such as circadian dysrhythmia, physical fatigue, illness, intoxication, dehydration, etc.

Fitness for Duty: Off-duty activities that negatively impact performance on the job such as the failure to adhere to sleep/rest requirements, alcohol restrictions, and other off-duty mandates.

> (Weigmann et al., 2023, p. 9; Human Factors Analysis and Classification System for Healthcare with useful categories with application to the Swiss Cheese Model of human factors).

In nursing, communication is one of what is known as the '6 C's', published in 2012 (NHS England, 2012). These values are care, compassion, competence, communication, courage, and commitment and became commonly referred to as the '6 C's of nursing'. There has recently been an addition of the '7 P's' of nursing': Protecting our planet; Prevention, protection, promotion, and reducing health inequalities; Person-centred practice; Public and patient safety; Professional leadership and integration; People and workforce development; and Professional culture (Devereux, 2023).

It could be argued that the '6 C's' are the professional behaviours expected of nurses and indeed all healthcare professionals as individuals, suggesting they are leadership attributes, whereas the '7 P's' are more about organisational principles and their culture, which would appear to be more about management. However, although both sets of values or principles explicitly or implicitly have patient care and safety at their core, the 7 P's state clearly that patient and public safety, along with 'professional leadership' merit specific identification as core principles. Thankfully, rather than replacing the 6 C's, it seems the 7 P's' are designed to work alongside them to bring about "better patient outcomes and creating a passionate, unstoppable nursing workforce" (Nurseplus, 2023).

These lists of behaviours and principles are applicable to all nurses and healthcare workers, however, according to Bennis (2022), there are six personal qualities that would enable an individual to become an effective and successful leader: Integrity, Dedication, Magnanimity, Humility, Openness, and Creativity, and although one would expect at least some of these qualities to be inherent in all nurses and healthcare workers, it is clear that not everyone has them all, for example, not everyone is creative. So according to Bennis, not everyone can become a leader.

Thinking Point

1 Is the statement that not everyone can become a leader true?
2 So, can anyone become a leader?
3 Are leaders born or made?

According to Leach (2021), the two predominant theories that leaders are either born or made are both true, despite citing research (Science Daily 2014) that suggests leadership is 30% genetic and 70% learned he goes on to say a person can be born with natural leadership abilities, and someone can learn how to be a good leader at work. Regardless of whether someone is a "born leader", everyone has room to learn new skills and grow in leadership competency. Whether leaders are born or made is a continuing moot point; however, what is clear is that leaders in healthcare are responsible and accountable for patient safety and therefore should receive the appropriate training, which, along with their experience, will equip them to provide the safest environment for those who have placed their trust in both the organisation and the individuals who work there to care and protect them to the highest standards.

Unfortunately, such responsibility and accountability is not always present in some organisations. There have been several high-profile cases where leadership was either inefficient or downright dangerous and, in some cases, led to the death of patients. Arguably one of the most well-known cases was that of the Mid Staffordshire Hospital scandal, mentioned earlier in the Chapter 2, comment made in the subsequent was that the need to "provide for a proper degree of accountability for senior managers and leaders to place all with responsibility for protecting the interests of patients on a level playing field". This comment is because of a number of observations made during the inquiry and subsequent report, such as the issue of 'whistleblowing' – "It is clear that a staff nurse's report in 2007 made a serious and substantial allegation about the leadership of A&E. This was not resolved by Trust management". The report is large, with many stories of neglect and lack of care and compassion, not least in nursing, where "As a result of poor leadership and staffing policies, a completely inadequate standard of nursing was offered on some wards at Stafford" (Francis, 2013, p. 45)

Sadly, despite the many positive changes in healthcare practice that this report fostered, it would appear that similar issues remain, for example, the death of a number of babies, reported in a BBC documentary entitled 'Midwives under Pressure' (BBC, 2024), where allegations of 'denial and deflection' are used if problems are reported and that 'senior managers and boards find it very difficult to admit that they have problems they don't know how to fix".

While mostly, if not all leadership failings are due, at least in part, to financial problems or staffing shortages or lack of other resources, these are not to be used as an excuse for poor leadership where patient safety and quality of care are compromised. History has many examples of exemplary leadership in dire situations, such as Shackelton's epic journey when he saved the lives of all 28 of his crew in one of the world's most extreme and hostile environments (Smith, 2020). Smith (2020) suggests that Shackelton's "greatest quality was that he put the welfare of his men above everything else". Leaders in healthcare would do well to follow his example and put the welfare of patients above everything else.

O'Brien states that "Change is a constant in life-maybe the only constant there is-and sudden change is not unusual" (O'Brien, 2015). The world is going through many transformative changes, particularly post-pandemic, and in healthcare, there is the constant need to control healthcare costs and overall to provide safety and "quality of care to all patients and clients" (Barr & Dowding, 2022). The ability to lead effectively during those changes, many of which are also driven by constant "government-legislation-induced change after change" (Barr & Dowding, 2022), is not simply the sign of a good and effective leader but what is required to provide safe and effective care for all. It is vital that all leaders, both present and future, take note of the theories related to leadership and the examples from history to guide them to provide some of the fundamental human needs Maslow (1943).

Organisational culture and patients' safety

As alluded to above, s2 HASAWA 1974 requires an employer to ensure appropriate systems of work and policies are in place. Likewise, employees owe patients a duty of care. This is to ensure that patients are not harmed by their (nurses') negligent actions or omissions. There is a corresponding professional requirement.

Management also has a common law duty of care to ensure that teams have the right skill-mix and patient-staff ratio. The recruitment and selection process includes an enhanced Disclosure Barring Service (DBS) check. This is a requirement for healthcare staff due to the fact they will be working with vulnerable people. This is the most in-depth DBS check to ensure protection of patients from potential criminals and possible harm. This record should include all spent and unspent convictions, cautions, and also reprimands and warnings. This should be seen as a fair and inclusive selection process. Appointment and promotion of staff should be down to merit and not favouritism or discrimination. Selection of staff based on 'fitting in' may result in discrimination or victimisation of potential patient advocates who may be subsequently targeted by managers as, 'troublemakers'. Staff are likely to be more productive if there is a positive atmosphere where they feel valued and listened to. A 'Speak up' culture should encourage staff to feel valued and raise concerns without fear of repercussions (Sir Robert Francis, 2015). If staff are happy and feel valued, they are more likely to demonstrate, productivity, dedication, and impacting patient safety.

A culture of openness with a two-way communication promoting a work-life balance should be a positive factor for promoting a safer environment for patient care. On the other hand, a toxic and culture of fear, without providing the staff appropriate resources, may result in negativity, poor attendance, and poor outcomes for patients. "A Populus poll for Mind, involving 2,060 adults in England and Wales in employment (polled between 6 and 10 March 2013) found that, while stress forced one in five workers to call in sick, 90 per cent say they lied to their boss about the real reason for not turning up" (Mind Resources, 2013).

Case Study: Police Investigating Dozens of Patient Deaths at Hospital in Brighton

Police are investigating dozens of deaths at the Royal Sussex County Hospital in Brighton over a five-year period, after two senior consultant surgeons who raised patient safety concerns were dismissed from their jobs.

Krishna Singh and Mansoor Foroughi are bringing employment tribunal claims against University Hospitals Sussex NHS Foundation Trust, which runs the hospital, after losing their jobs. Singh, a general surgeon, was clinical director for abdominal surgery and medicine, and Foroughi, a neurosurgeon, specialises in brain and spine surgery.

The *Guardian*, which broke the story, reported that the number of deaths is around 40. A statement from Sussex Police said that the force had "received allegations of medical negligence at the Royal Sussex County Hospital, Brighton, and is currently assessing these allegations".

(Dyer, 2023, p. 1356)

Thinking Point

1 While respecting confidentiality, please reflect on potential causes of an under resourced work environment.
2 What are the likely causes and potential adverse results?
3 If you had concerns, what measures are open to you in your organisation that you would take in order to ensure that the situation is remedied if you permanently have inadequate (human and material) resources.

Clearly dangerous and risky practice can easily be become the norm or accepted way within the culture of an organisation. Inadequate staffing levels, for example, may result in poor or inadequate risk assessment and risk management with evaluation or reviewer of interventions and inevitably harm to patients. The Francis Report (2013) found that,

There was an unacceptable delay in addressing the issue of shortage of skilled nursing staff...

The result was both to deprive the hospital of a proper level of nursing staff and provide a healthier picture of the situation of the financial health of the Trust than the true reality, healthy finances being material in the achievement of Foundation Trust status. While the system appeared to pay lip service to the need not to compromise services and their quality, it is remarkable how little attention was paid to the potential impact of proposed savings on quality and safety.

(Francis Report)

A toxic culture may consequently be embedded in organisations where no one cares about advocacy or safeguarding vulnerable patients of healthcare providers resulting in negative impact on the health service users. One recent example is outlined below:

Case Study: UK National Scandal: 20,000 Mental Health Patients 'Raped, Sexually Assaulted' in NHS Care (January 2024)

A new investigation revealed that tens of thousands of mental health patients have been raped, sexually abused, assaulted, or harassed while being treated in UK's National Health Service (NHS) mental hospitals, in what is described as a 'national scandal'. The joint investigation carried out by The Independent and Sky News and run-on Sunday, uncovered nearly 20,000 'sexual safety incidents', involving both patients and staff, across more than 30 mental health trusts in England between 2019 and 2023.

The report defines sexual safety incidents as 'any unwanted sexual behaviour that makes a person feel uncomfortable or unsafe. This includes rape, sexual assault, sexual harassment, comments of a sexual nature, or observing sexual behaviour, including exposure to nakedness'.

Nearly 4,000 sexual safety incidents were reported between January and August 2023 – higher than the annual total for both 2019 and 2020, the investigation revealed following more than 50 freedom of information requests to NHS England mental health trusts.

A separate freedom of information request conducted by *The Independent* also revealed out of more than 800 allegations of sexual assault and rape involving female patients across more than 20 trusts between 2019 and 2023, only 95 were reported to the police.

Former Victim's Commissioner Dame Vera Baird has said the findings are a 'national scandal'.

(Press TV, 2024, https://www.presstv.ir/Detail/2024/01/29/719088/UK-Conservatives-Mental-Health-Patients-Sexual-Abuse-NHS)

Unsafe actions

The culture of an organisation may help meeting patient outcomes and determine a healthy working environment. The quality of the working relationship between a given organisation's management and the staff working for them should be at the heart of the quality of care. The Chartered Institute of Personnel Development (CIPD, 2022) defines the employee relationship as '… transactional…and the relationships are shaped by the bargaining power of the parties, and in most cases, this is unequal, with the employer enjoying the more powerful position' (Bennett et al. 2020, p. 17).

Examples of contributory factors to decision-making are due to human factors as communication is crucial and plays a part in human factors, for example, decision-making with lack of or poor communication or skill-based errors' poor (Wiegmann 2023). Other areas of concern are 'skill-based' or perceptual errors which may result in human perceptions as well as 'bending the rules'.

A landmark case showed examples of miscommunication issues (please also see Chapter 2) in a healthcare situation sadly led to a patient's death and is provided below:

Case Study: Bromiley Case, Parliamentary Committee on Health Report

Elaine Bromiley went into hospital for a routine sinus operation and during anaesthetic induction, it all went horribly wrong. Her airway obstructed and the team was unable to gain a secure airway. For 20 minutes, they attempted to achieve a stable airway, during which time her oxygen saturations were around 40%. Although she survived, she sustained serious hypoxic brain injury and 13 days later her life support was turned off. Martin (her husband) was an airline pilot with an interest in human factors and he subsequently formed the Clinical Human Factors Group in 2007. One of the main teamwork lessons from Elaine's case was communication. Communication between team members is crucial, and in Elaine's case, the communication process dried up completely. There were three senior and experienced doctors in the room – two anaesthetic consultants and an ENT consultant. They did not communicate with each other, and nobody actually vocalised what was happening (i.e., this patient is in trouble, this is a 'can't intubate, can't ventilate' situation).

(Select Committee on Health Written Evidence, Memorandum by the Clinical Human Factors Group (CHFG) (PS 24), 2008)

Subject to vicarious liability, the employer stands to benefit from the positive actions of employees and, likewise, must be held to account for the negative actions of their employees. This is subject to the doctrine of 'respondeat superior', which means that the employer is liable, and the employees are exempted from penalties provided employees are following the employee policy.

Case Law: Weddall v Barchester Healthcare Ltd [2012] EWCA Civ 25

Mr Weddall was a deputy manager at a care home. One evening while on duty, Mr Weddall telephoned Mr Marsh, a senior health assistant, who was off duty and asked him if he was willing to work a nightshift as another employee had turned in sick.

Mr Marsh was very drunk and became angry and upset on the call, as he thought Mr Weddall was mocking him. Twenty minutes later, Mr Marsh cycled to the care home and (hopping mad) violently attacked Mr Weddall. Mr Marsh was sentenced to 15 months imprisonment for a criminal assault. Mr Weddall brought a claim against Barchester Homes, alleging that it was vicariously liable for Mr Marsh's actions.

- The Appeal Court found that Mr Marsh's actions were "an independent venture ... separate and distinct from Marsh's employment as a Senior Health Assistant at a care home".

NHS organisations are indemnified by the NHS Resolution, and they will be required to pay an insurance premium towards insuring their healthcare provision activities.

Additionally, healthcare professionals are also required to indemnify their own practice, subject to the Health Care and Associated Professions (Indemnity Arrangements) Order 2014.

Staff wellbeing, safety and liability

Healthcare professional codes of conduct also require staff to follow the above legal standard of care. All staff must ensure they have received up-to-date training on technique and use of any equipment.

HASAWA 1974, Section 7

a To take reasonable care for the health and safety of himself and others who may be affected by his acts or omissions at work.
b To co-operate with his employer or any other person, so far as is necessary.

Clinical governance, as outlined in Chapter 2 on the seven pillars, defines the concept of quality of care in the provision of healthcare services, inevitably subject to human factors related to management and staff. Organisational cultures may affect patient outcomes. Human factors may unfortunately adversely have a knock-on effect on the quality of healthcare delivery. All healthcare providers must also ensure that they have a well-resourced, effective, positive, and well-resourced environment. Clinical governance defines the wellbeing of staff and a healthy work environment which is embedded in positive industrial relations. A healthy working environment includes appropriate staff-patient ratios.

More recently, in comparable western countries including the UK, healthcare staff have been under more pressure due to working in stressful conditions, with recruitment issues, especially during the COVID pandemic. This in turn has impacted on patient safety. There was evidence of 'a substantial number of staff sickness especially in mental health services, with a projected increase in absenteeism of 70% on staff' and 52% strongly agreeing to concerns about staff wellbeing and 41% NHS Providers and only 1% strongly disagreeing (CIPD, 2022). The Kings Fund (2023) also acknowledged staff shortage across the NHS, since during the first lockdown in March 2020. In September 2023, the overall NHS vacancy rate was 8.4%, or 121,000 full-time equivalent (FTE) roles. In 2022/23, the overall social care vacancy rate was 9.9% or 152,000 roles. This had inevitably a knock-on effect on patient safety due to staff shortages or staff who were stressed out. The RCN (2021) Employment survey report on workforce experience found that staff have increasingly been on the receiving end of abuse, with 64.3% admitting that they had experienced abuse from patient service use and relative in the previous 12 months, including 26% reporting physical violence. Black and ethnic minority staff were more likely to be victims.

Abuse of staff may negatively affect impact their performance with a negative impact on patient wellbeing. This means that staff are more likely to go off sick or to leave their jobs with stress related illnesses as a result, the added pressure may impact on patient safety. Office of National Statistics (ONS) in 2017 identified female nurses as having a risk of suicide 23% above the risk in women in other occupations. According to the National Confidential Inquiry into Suicide and Safety in Mental Health (NCISH, 2020), it found that of 281 nurses who died by suicide over the six-year study period: of these 204 (73%) were female – this was the focus of the study.

Case Study: University Hospitals Birmingham, Half of staff felt bullied.

The findings come from an independent review commissioned by University Hospitals Birmingham (UHB) NHS Trust.

It has been at the centre of NHS scrutiny after a culture of fear was uncovered in a BBC Newsnight investigation.

UHB has apologised for 'unacceptable behaviours'.

It added it was committed to changing the working environment.

The trust is one of the largest of its kind in England, responsible for the Queen Elizabeth (QE), Heartlands, Good Hope and Solihull hospitals, as well as some community services.

Of 2,884 respondents to a staff survey, 53% said they had felt bullied or harassed at work, while only 16% believed their concerns would be taken up by their employer.

Many said they were fearful to complain "as they believed it could worsen the situation", the review team found.

(https://www.bbc.co.uk/news/uk-england-birmingham-66936628)

- Female nurses were older than other women who died by suicide; nearly half were aged 45–54 years (N = 87, 43%).
- The most common method of suicide for female nurses was self-poisoning (42%).
- More than half (60%) of female nurses who died were not in contact with mental health services.

(NCISH, 2020, https://documents.manchester.ac.uk/display.aspx?DocID=49577)

The NMC annual survey also found that the feedback from staff who left the register was at times negative, for example,

I've enjoyed my career in the NHS and as a community nurse, but I'm unsure if I would recommend this career as the stress and pressure on nurses this day is almost intolerable. "Nurse, England, aged 65+".

(NMC, 2023, https://www.nmc.org.uk/globalassets/sitedocuments/data-reports/may-2023/annual-data-report-leavers-survey-2023.pdf)

The employer-employee relationship is contractual, under the Advisory Conciliation and Arbitration Service (ACAS) Code of Practice on grievance and disciplinary procedures (2015), subject to s 199 of the Trade Union and Labour Relations (Consolidation) Act (1992). ACAS is publicly funded. Healthcare professionals must advocate for vulnerable patients and service users. They are also supported by their union or employer appointed workplace representatives.

The practice of derogation to maintain local minimum levels had lacked certainty, with limited effect. Voluntary agreements between employer and employee representatives aim to ensure that there are minimum levels of staff agreed. This may or may not have worked depending on local industrial agreements. One example was, during the junior doctors' strike in August 2023, when the British Medical Association (BMA) refused 17 applications for derogations where both local clinical leaders and their own local representatives had agreed it was necessary and reasonable to keep patients safe. The law has since changed when section 234F of that act updated the Trade Union and Labour Relations (Consolidation) Act 1992, by introducing a requirement for unions to give notice to employers of industrial action.

(1) An act done by a trade union to induce a person to take part, or continue to take part, in industrial action is not protected as respects his employer unless

the union has taken or takes such steps as are reasonably necessary to ensure that the employer receives within the appropriate period a relevant notice covering the act.

Since November 2023, the enactment of the Strikes (Minimum Service Levels) Act 2023 is a UK wide statute. The Scottish Government, nevertheless, will not enforce it. This means that minimum service is required in order to provide minimum services. The question is may be defining what is agreed as 'minimum'. In practice, most unions will have local arrangements with their local management. The secretary of state must decide the minimum levels which must be provided during strikes for each sector. Section 234B of the above statute applies to key service providers such as

a health services,
b fire and rescue services,
c education services,
d transport services,
e decommissioning of nuclear installations and management of radioactive waste and spent fuel, and
f border security.

(Strikes (Minimum Service Levels) Act 2023)

Conclusion

Despite the legal framework, policies, theories, publications, real life case studies, and case law examples, some of which have been included above, more needs to be done to raise awareness and to keep staff informed. Organisational cultures, management, and individual decisions matter. Organisations, everyone in a management role as well as clinicians delivering care, should themselves be informed and reminded of their duties and responsibilities. On patient safety, the first tenet for all healthcare professionals should be 'to do no harm' and a safe environment when caring for patients (in all categories of care) when working with patients, colleagues, loved ones, and employees.

Hopefully, this chapter will have also provided the reader with an opportunity for application and reflection on key management and leadership theory, considering issues which have been raised above. This should also be a stark reminder of what could happen if organisations, management, and staff do not prioritise patients' needs in everything and if they do not prioritise safe delivery of care.

References

Aasland MS, Skogstad A, Notelaers G. *et al* (2009) The prevalence of destructive leadership, *BJM*, 21(2), 438–452, https://onlinelibrary.wiley.com/doi/abs/10.1111/j.1467-8551.2009.00672.x

ACAS (2015) Available online at: https://www.acas.org.uk/acas-code-of-practice-on-disciplinary-and-grievance-procedures (Accessed on 2nd February 2024)

Barr J, Dowding L (2022) Leadership in healthcare London. SAGE Publications

BBC Panorama (2024) Midwives under pressure, Available online at: https://www.bbc.co.uk/iplayer/episode/m001vw4n/panorama-midwives-under-pressure (Accessed on 5th March 2024)

Belbin M (1981) Belbin team roles, Available online at: https://www.belbin.com/about/belbin-team-roles (Accessed on 5th March 2024)

Bennett T, Saundry R, Virginia Fisher V (2020) Managing employment relations, Available online at: https://www.koganpage.com/hr-learning-development/managing-employment-relations-9781789661453 (Accessed on 5th January 2024)

Bennis W (2022) Six personal qualities of leadership, Available online at: https://www.linkedin.com/pulse/six-personal-qualities-leadership-warren-/?utm_source=share&utm_medium=member_android&utm_campaign=share_via (Accessed on 5th March 2024)

Bennis WG, Nanus B (2012) Leaders: Strategies for taking charge (2nd ed). New York: Harper Collins

Cambridge Dictionary (no date) Available online at: https://dictionary.cambridge.org/dictionary/english/manage (Accessed on 5th March 2024)

Chartered Institute of Personnel Development (2022) Fact sheet, health and wellbeing at work, Available online at: https://www.cipd.org/uk/knowledge/factsheets/relations-employees-factsheet/ (Accessed on 2nd February 2024)

Chartered Institute of Personnel Development Health and Wellbeing at Work, Available online at: https://www.cipd.org/globalassets/media/comms/news/ahealth-wellbeing-work-report-2022_tcm18-108440.pdf (Accessed on 3rd February 2024)

Daft RL (2017) The leadership experience (6th ed). Delhi: Centage

DePree M (2004) [1987] Leadership is an art. New York: Doubleday

Devereux E (2023) New 7Ps for nursing unveiled as part of CNO strategy, Nursing Times (Accessed on 5th March 2024)

Dyer C (2023) Case Study: Police investigating dozens of patient deaths at hospital in Brighton, *BMJ*, 381, 1356

Evesson J, Oxenbridge S (2015) Seeking better solutions: Tackling bullying and ill-treatment in Britain's workplaces, Available online at: https://www.diversitymckenzie.co.uk/wp-content/uploads/2016/07/Seeking-better-solutions-tackling-bullying-and-ill-treatment-in-Britains-workplaces.pdf (Accessed on 5th March 2024)

Flint J (2023) What is the key difference between a manager and a leader? Available online at: https://www.salford.ac.uk/spd/what-key-difference-between-manager-and-leader (Accessed on 5th March 2024)

Francis R (2013) Report of the Mid Staffordshire NHS Foundation (2013). Executive summary, Available online at: https://assets.publishing.service.gov.uk/media/5a7ba0faed915d13110607c8/0947.pdf (Accessed on 5th March 2024)

Health and Safety Department (2022) Available online at: https://www.hsdept.co.uk/services/health-safety-policies-procedure/employers-responsibilities-for-health-and-safety/ (Accessed on 5th March 2024)

Health and Safety Executive (1974) Health and safety at work act, Available online at: https://www.hse.gov.uk/legislation/hswa.htm (Accessed on 5th March 2024)

Health and Social Care Act (2012) Available online at: https://www.legislation.gov.uk/ukpga/2012/7/contents/enacted (Accessed on 24th May 2024)

Health Care and Associated Professions (Indemnity Arrangements) Order 2014

Kings Fund (2023) Staff Shortages. Available online at: https://www.kingsfund.org.uk/insight-and-analysis/data-and-charts/staff-shortages#:~:text=This%20shortage%20in%20staff%20can,9.9%25%2C%20or%20152%2C000%20roles (Accessed on 24th May 2024)

Kline R (2019) Leadership in the NHS, BJM Leader, Available online at: https://web.archive.org/web/20220922052110id_/https://bmjleader.bmj.com/content/leader/early/2022/09/11/leader-2022-000622.full.pdf (Accessed on 24th May 2024)

Leach B (2021) Born leaders vs. made leaders: Are leaders born or trained? Available online at: https://unboxedtechnology.com/blog/difference-between-born-leader-and-made-leader/#:~:text=to%20your%20employees.,Are%20Leaders%20Born%20or%20Trained%3F,%25%20genetic%20and%2070%25%20learned (Accessed on 5th March 2024).

Leech D (2019) Available online at: https://www.nationalhealthexecutive.com/articles/leadership-and-management-are-two-different-roles-what-your-job-really (Accessed on 5th March 2024)

Maslow AH (1943) A theory of human motivation, Psychol Rev, 50(4), 370–396

National Confidential Inquiry into Suicide and Safety in Mental Health (NCISH) (2020). Suicide by female nurses: A brief report, University of Manchester, Available online at: https://documents.manchester.ac.uk/display.aspx?DocID=49577 (Accessed on 4th January 2024)

NHS England (2012) Available online at: https://www.england.nhs.uk/wp-content/uploads/2012/12/compassion-in-practice.pdf (Accessed on 5th March 2024)

NMC (2023) Annual Data Reports, Available online at: https://www.nmc.org.uk/globalassets/sitedocuments/data-reports/may-2023/annual-data-report-leavers-survey-2023.pdf (Accessed on 35th May 2024)

Nurseplus (2023) The new 7 P's of nursing, Available online at: https://www.nurseplusuk.com/blog/2023/12/the-new-7-Ps-of-nursing (Accessed on 5th March 2024)

O'Brien P (2015) Great decisions, perfect timing: Cultivating intuitive intelligence. Portland Oregon Divination Foundation Press.

Press TV (2024) Available online at: https://www.presstv.ir/Detail/2024/01/29/719088/UK-Conservatives-Mental-Health-Patients-Sexual-Abuse-NHS (Accessed on 5th February 2024)

RCN (2021) Employment survey report 2021: Workforce diversity and employment experiences, Available online at: https://www.rcn.org.uk/Professional-Development/publications/employment-survey-report-2021-uk-pub-010-216 (Accessed on 4th January 2024)

RCN (2024) Leadership skills: How to demonstrate and develop leadership skills within your career, Available online at: https://www.rcn.org.uk/Professional-Development/Your-career/Nurse/Leadership-skills (Accessed on 24th May 2024)

Science Daily (2014) Available online at: https://www.sciencedaily.com/releases/2014/10/141006133228.htm (Accessed on 5th March 2024).

Sir Robert Francis' Freedom to Speak Up review (2015) Available online at: https://www.gov.uk/government/publications/sir-robert-francis-freedom-to-speak-up-review (Accessed on 24th May 2024)

Smith M (2020) Shackleton, Available online at: https://shackleton.com/blogs/articles/shackleton-great-leader (Accessed on 5th March 2024).

Strikes (Minimum Service Levels) Act (2023) Available online at: https://www.legislation.gov.uk/ukpga/2023/39/enacted (Accessed on 25th May 2024)

Trade Union and Labour Relations (Consolidation) Act (1992), s 199.

Weddall v Barchester Healthcare Ltd [2012] EWCA Civ 25.

Weigmann DA, Wood LJ, Cohen TN, Shappell SA (2023) Understanding the "Swiss Cheese Model" and its application to patient safety, Available online at: https://www.ncbi.nlm.nih.gov/pmc/articles/PMC8514562/ (Accessed on 5th March 2024)

8 Delivering safe end-of-life care

Cheyne Truman and Paul Buka

Introduction

Defining and understanding end-of-life and palliative care are important aspects of any health care professional's (HCP) role. It would be remiss to not draw attention to the concepts of decision-making and safe practice therein, having had substantial experience in caring for those nearing their end-of-life and on palliative care pathways. While end-of-life and palliative care come with their own challenges for HCPs and carers, it is vital that shared decision-making, irrespective of the challenges for all involved, is paramount and focussed on the patient's wellbeing and safety.

This chapter will focus on end-of-life care, though 'palliative' care is included, but some overlap is inevitable and context is provided. Elements of this very nature of care have often been found to have both positive and negative impacts on quality of care, person-centred outcomes and the wellbeing of those supporting the individual in whatever capacity. Moreover, ethical dilemmas that frequently pose difficulties for clinicians, carers and loved ones and how decisions are made for patients, with patients and all the while managing our own individual beliefs, emotions and desires and needs of the patient will be considered. To help manage this complicated and valuable area of care, there is much policy, legislation, process and guidance, which will be explored further in this chapter. Also explored will be the more personal impact on individuals within this care circle while also drawing upon some of individual authors' own experiences. All identifying details will be anonymised and pseudonyms used.

End-of-life and palliative care: historical context

Post-war, the inception of the UK welfare state and the National Health Service (NHS, 1948) pledged to provide safe care from 'cradle to grave'; however, for the first two decades little evidence exists in the NHS regarding any guidance for care of dying patients (Clark, 2014). Furthermore, Clark (2014) introduces two key reports populated by external sources from the 1950s. One such report was born out of a survey in Great Britain and Northern Ireland assessing needs of domiciliary care for those with cancer, which found patients were receiving treatment or care too late, were 'gravely ill', or bedbound. This report also highlighted the physical, social and impact on mental health

DOI: 10.4324/9781003376934-8

for these 7050 cases, with a variety of recommendations cited, including care provision strategies, information, and equipment. Furthermore, Clark (2014) summarises the second report, 'Peace at the Last' by Brigadier Glyn Hughes, which was created in 1960 and found that terminal care, though preferred to be at home, was insufficient in the NHS and was predominantly provided by charitable and religious organisations, and volunteers in part due to infrastructure, financial burden, staffing and expertise required. He also surmised that a large proportion of people needing expert terminal care were dying outside of the NHS. What came next was of significance in end-of-life and palliative care. This was the creation of St. Christopher's Hospice UK, emanating from the modern hospice movement orchestrated by Saunders (1967), a pioneering nurse who paved the way for dignified and sensitive hospice care as it is today. She also presented a framework regarding pain management of the dying person to include physical, psychological, social and spiritual considerations, 'total pain' theory, contributing to a dignified death and quality of life. It was not, however, until 2014 that the World Health Organization (WHO) called for a global improvement of access, guidelines, tools and delivery of palliative care at the core of health provision (WHO, 2020).

Defining end-of-life care or palliative care?

Marie Curie defined end-of-life care as that which 'involves treatment, care and support for people who are thought to be in the last year of life' (Marie Curie, 2022a). However, the NHS would include those in the last year of their life (NHS, 2023). The WHO (2020) discusses palliative care as 'improving the quality of life for patients and that of their families who faced challenges associated with lighter illness whether physical psychological social or spiritual. The quality of my caregivers improves as well'. Palliative care, on the other hand according to Marie Curie (2022b), can include and is broader than end-of-life and 'offers physical, emotional and practical support for people with a terminal diagnosis'. Furthermore, palliative care can be offered at any time post-diagnosis. More recently (NICE, 2023) defines palliative care as 'active holistic care of patients and other symptoms and provision of psychological, social and spiritual support'. It is important therefore to understand that while these terms are often used interchangeably, they are different, but this separation does not negate the patient safety and shared decision-making requirements for effective care.

Ethico-legal perspectives

End-of-life care must be the most important aspect of decision-making for patients or service users. Decisions should be patient-centred NHS Constitution (2013) and for their welfare and safety, which is paramount in decision-making. While following national guidelines, clinicians' decision-making should be subject to the legal and ethical framework for decision-making with implications for patients' safety and their human rights. Individual 'liberty' or freedom to make decisions has been contended by ethicists such as JS Mill's (1806–1873). Utilitarianism proponents advocated individual right to take their own lives, provided that no other person suffers directly as a result (Philp, 2015). Other moral philosophers like Emmanuel Kant (1724–1804) justified suicide based on the 'categorical imperative' or unconditional moral obligation in his deontology moral principle, which is binding in all circumstances (Robson, 2021). The problem is that this is subjective and may be very difficult to justify.

Ethical dilemmas on decision-making may arise due to a conflict of interests, i.e., that of the patient versus those of the loved ones, vis-a-vis clinicians and/or society at large. This is at the heart of Biomedical ethics or Bioethics principles, expressed by Beauchamp and Childress (2019) as respect for autonomy, nonmaleficence, beneficence and justice. Patient safety is at the focus of the 'To do no harm' moral principle.

Fairness and autonomy are also applicable when it comes to resources and patient-centred decision-making. Subject to the European Convention on Human Rights (ECHR, 1950a), Article 2 defines the right to life.

> Everyone's right to life shall be protected by law. No one shall be deprived of his life intentionally save in the execution of a sentence of a court following his conviction of a crime for which the penalty is provided by law.
> (https://www.equalityhumanrights.com/en/human-rights-act/article-2-right-life#:~:text=Everyone's%20 right%20to%20life%20shall,2)

A 'living will' is in fact an Advance Directive or Advance Decision to refuse treatment (ADRT), which are legally binding. The most common example is a person's wishes to refuse treatment or to not be resuscitated in the event of a cardiac arrest.

Furthermore, an Advance Statement is an indication or personal preferences or wishes and is not legally binding and less formal. This could be an expression of a person's wishes which should be considered when care planning, for example, where they would like to spend their last days. This does not need to be in writing.

A patient may also officially appoint another trusted individual, Lasting Power of Attorney (LPA) to make decisions on their behalf. Prior to obtaining consent, they should be fully informed of the benefits and consequences of refusing treatment. The consent must be written, with a witnessed signing.

Case Law C (Adult, Refusal of Treatment) [1994] 1 All ER 819

Mental illness and a patient's capacity.

C diagnosed with paranoid schizophrenia and was detained in Broadmoor secure hospital. He developed gangrene in his leg but against medical advice, refused to consent to an amputation.

The Court upheld C's decision.

Legal Principle: The fact that a person has a mental illness does not automatically mean they lack capacity to make a decision about medical treatment.

Patients who have capacity can make their own decisions to refuse treatment, even if those decisions appear irrational to the doctor or may place the patient's health or their life at risk.

(http://www.gmc-uk.org/guidance/ethical_guidance/consent_guidance_common_law.asp)

National frameworks

Frameworks affecting end-of-life care have evolved over time, for legal reasons and as lessons are learnt. One such example includes 'Ambitions for palliative and end-of-life care' (National Palliative and End-of-Life Care Partnership, 2021). The key objective of this framework is to achieve individualised care of the dying person while encompassing the needs of carers, families and those of importance to the dying person, not excluding the bereaved. Nationally, each death must matter, whether sudden, gradual or unexpected. Death does and will affect 100% of the nation. Six ambitions were developed, namely, 'Each person is seen as an individual, each person gets access to fair care, maximising comfort and wellbeing, care is coordinated, all staff are prepared to care and each community is prepared to care'. What does this mean in reality? It means education and training is paramount for staff, carers and the communities. Support, information and personalised care planning are just some of the priority foundations of effective end-of-life care.

The NHS Long Term Plan (2019) also explored the need for individuals to have greater control of their own care and that it be personalised, with shared decision-making, from 'maternity to end-of-life'. Additionally, the Gold Standards Framework (2023), which stipulates that 'Everyone deserves Gold Standard end-of-life care', seeks to achieve this through evidence-based training, education and guidance, irrespective of the setting. The Cross Boundary Care (CBC) approach seeks to achieve a population approach to end-of-life care for those in their final year/s by promoting integrated care across all services to meet individual's wishes and support them to live and die well. CBC training is in its early stages but is already seeing significantly improved integration across settings, in key sites around the country and internationally. The Proactive Identification Guidance tool is being used to support clinicians in early detection of decline in the dying person, therefore enabling improved assessments, care planning, decision-making and meeting individual needs and wishes.

Decision-making framework and healthcare multidisciplinary teams

The General Medical Council (GMC) shares good practice and decision-making models across service boundaries that consider mental capacity or lack thereof, roles of those close to the patient, clinical judgements and emotional challenges in end-of-life decision-making. Essentially, of paramount importance should be the patient, their wishes, needs and quality care. Decision-makers should include a variety of appropriate medical and healthcare professionals, the patient and those they 'want' to be involved. Furthermore, confidentiality and appropriate sharing of information is governed firmly by the law and policy regulations.

Careful consideration must be given to the healthcare professionals who have a duty of confidentiality to protect confidential patient information (Data Protection Act 2018): Examples are Access to Health Records Act (1990) (England, Scotland, and Wales), Access to Health Records (Northern Ireland) Order (1993), Data Protection Act (2018), Adult Support and Protection (Scotland) Act (2007) and Care

Act (2014). Despite the legalities of information sharing, multi-disciplinary working is key to quality end-of-life care and treatment. The across-service boundaries aspect of shared decision-making must not be forgotten due to complexities of sharing information, because without this shared decision-making, patient safety is inevitably compromised. Making sound clinical judgements in end-of-life and palliative care cannot be made intrinsically by any one individual, though the one individual at the centre is the patient. This must not change if their safety is to be maintained.

Equally, the emotional challenges that come with this decision-making ought to be considered at every stage of the clinical reasoning, decision-making, withdrawal of treatment, postponement or implementation to shift the focus of care to comfort and dignity. These emotional challenges apply to patients, those close to them and healthcare professionals involved.

When using unbiased clinical judgement in decision-making at end-of-life or palliative care, there is a constant need to weigh up benefits, burdens and risks, whatever trajectory the decision-making will take. Consent and best interests must be discussed at every step, because it is not enough to decide treatment on clinical grounds while disputing best interests or patients' wishes without considering the implications of that decision irrespective of the anticipated outcome. No matter the best interests, risks or benefits, without consent, patient safety is at risk.

A patient may make an advance decision or directive, which is valid, provided they have the mental capacity at the time of making that decision, under the Mental Capacity Act (2005), sections 1 and 2. This means that the decision must be clear and unambiguous, applicable to persons above the age of 18. This does not apply to individuals who lack capacity to make their own decisions; others with the power of attorney may make decision on their behalf. The Court of Protection may also be asked to intervene and advocate for patients who lack capacity to make decisions or where there are disagreements between stakeholders. It is worth noting that often patients at end-of-life lose capacity due to unconsciousness or may experience fluctuating capacity. Equally, those with brain disease would also lose not only physical but also mental capacity, and healthcare professionals would complete a best interest decision under the Mental Capacity Act (2005).

The timing of discussions regarding future care, though voluntary, is paramount and should happen early in the disease stages, if time allows, as part of advance care planning. By having these discussions early prevents confusion later, when carers and healthcare professionals do not know the wishes of the patient. It is not ideal or dignified to have this discussion in times of crisis. Some patients may not wish to discuss advance care planning. Healthcare professionals may feel the discomfort of the person when they need to have such difficult conversations.

The Care Quality Commission (2022), Royal Pharmaceutical Society (2019), National Institute for Health and Care Excellence (2015) and GMC (2021) all provide guidance policies and regulations regarding safe prescription and administration of medications and treatment therapies, which healthcare teams must follow. End-of-life decision-making includes but is not limited to controlled drugs and antipsychotics with multiple uses such as haloperidol, which is often used across mental health and in end-of-life for differing purposes. Contraindications and side effects must be considered carefully, as well as underlying existing medical conditions. In end-of-life care, however, the benefits that outweigh existing harms or risks tend to be an overriding medical consideration to achieve patient comfort (Cadogan et al., 2021) (see Chapter 5 on medicines management). It is important to note that the COVID-19 pandemic saw many challenges, emergency standards and circumstances that impeded the development, achievement and adherence to these frameworks. See the scenario below:

Case Scenario: COVID-19 PANDEMIC Visits Restrictions, One Prebooked per Patient for 1 hr per day

A newly registered nurse (NRN) caring for a terminally ill gentleman in his 50s, in hospital. He had three children of varying ages, a spouse and parents who lived locally.

Thanks to the GSF Framework's Proactive Identification Guidance Tool, clinicians were able to ascertain that this gentleman was likely nearing the end of his life within weeks to days (an estimation based on clinical evidence and investigations).

Sadly, the NRN had instructions to advise his spouse to choose one of their children to visit for an hour per day. Permission had been granted for his spouse to be present during the visits.

This discussion was challenging and emotive for all, and his spouse asked all the anticipated questions regarding discharge, care in the community, hospice bed, hospice at home and private care at home.

In consideration of the frameworks noted above, meeting these needs and wishes should have been priority especially as he wanted to die at home with his family.

COVID-19 rules and regulations at the time made this impossible. Drawing upon the expertise of other speciality teams like the palliative specialist nurses, social workers and care agencies, enquiries were made. The family also made all their own enquiries, but because he was safe, in a hospital bed, with healthcare available 24/7, he could not be moved due to lack of care options available outside of the hospital.

There was no real solution other than what was achieved on what was believed to be his last day, when arrangements were made for his spouse and three children to be with him at his side for his final hours. Staff were also able to make an allowance for his parents to visit for an hour, but without the other family members in the room.

While we could not meet his wishes of dying at home, healthcare staff were at least able to work together to enable his family to be at his bedside in his last hours.

Thinking Point

1   Was patient safety the deciding factor over patient choice and needs?
2   Did patient safety concerns hinder quality of care?
3   Did this affect adherence to legal frameworks and policies? If so, which ones? Which should have been prioritised?
4   How do you feel about the decision-making that occurred in this scenario?

Across borders: a brief outline of comparative analysis of physician-assisted suicide

Ethics or bioethics informs international legal frameworks. Tensions between preservation of life and 'sanctity of life' versus 'the right to die' are inevitable. Passive euthanasia amounts to the withdrawal of treatment or nutrition as in the Tony Bland (1993) case. This is justifiable in some instances.

There is a clear distinction between palliative care and physician-assisted suicide. The latter, being 'active', is legal in a few countries. This fact could be a 'slippery slope'. Long-established pro-physician-assisted euthanasia practicing countries include Switzerland, Southwestern Australia and Oregon, USA, which have long been advocates. Some concerns on motives have emerged with '…three most frequently mentioned end-of-life concerns (*being*), loss of autonomy (89.5%), decreasing ability to participate in activities that made life enjoyable (89.5%), and loss of dignity (65.4%) (Public Health Oregon, 2017, p. 6). Other countries which have followed suit are all Australian states, New Zealand, a handful USA states such as Washington and California as well as Canada, which has seen a rise of 30% in assisted suicide cases since the implementation of legislation CBC News (2023). European countries where this is permissible are Belgium and Luxembourg. Examples of countries which have recently shielded away from euthanasia are UK as well as France.

Pro-euthanasia systems which legitimise physician-assisted suicide are broadly similar, though most would allow euthanasia for incurable disease and/or those in unbearable pain as well as the patient's mental capacity for making the choice.

Wrongful life, right to die: PVS decisions and patient safety

This aspect is related to the right to die; voluntary euthanasia will be addressed below. Best interests may also be relevant where a person lacks capacity and the Court of Protection may determine rights in the best interests, for example, patients in persistent vegetative state (PVS). The patient's human right to informed consent is at the heart of decision-making. They have a right to refuse treatment, which may be seen as an 'unwise' decision (and which may put them at risk). The Court of Protection may decide the 'best interests' on behalf of a patient who lacks capacity.

Thomas Aquinas' (1225–1274) 'double effect' theory, which justifies the administration of narcotic medications for pain relief, is permissible if aim is pain control, nevertheless hastening the death of a patient. Countries such as Switzerland continue to be hosts to UK nationals who choose to travel for the purpose of humanely ending their lives there. It should be noted that anyone accompanying another for physician-assisted suicide with the purpose of 'humanely' ending their lives may be prosecuted for aiding and abetting.

Subject to s1, Suicide Act (1961), suicide is no longer a crime. Under sections 2 and 3 of the same statute, however, it remains a criminal offence for a third party, including clinicians, to '…aid and abet', and this includes assisting or encouraging another to commit suicide, which is punishable by up to 14 years in prison. This includes clinicians. The Suicide Act 1961 is related to autonomy and the individual right to choose. Before 1961, suicide was a crime. Since 1961 it has not been a crime under the Suicide Act 1961, sections 2 and 3; nevertheless, assisting is. Relevant parts of the change in the law are:

Section 2

A person who aids, abets, counsels, or procures the suicide of another, or an attempt by another to commit suicide, shall be liable on conviction on indictment to imprisonment for a term not exceeding fourteen years.

Section 3

If on the trial of an indictment for murder or manslaughter it is proved that the accused aided, abetted, counselled or procured suicide of the person in question, the jury may find him/her guilty of that offence.

The classification of euthanasia is active where positive steps are taken to end life and/or *passive* where treatment or life-sustaining measures are withdrawn.

A patient who is deemed to have capacity, however, as in the *Re C (Adult, refusal of treatment) [1994] 1 All ER 819*may refuse treatment even if this means risking their own life. This case established the principle that if a person's capacity is established, they have a right to make a decision which may adversely affect them or put their life at risk. Ethical dilemmas may arise on withdrawal of treatment if a person lacks capacity, such as children or frail persons in a PVS.

Case Law: Airedale NHS Trust v Bland [1993] AC 789

Following the Hillsborough disaster, Tony Bland was in a PSV and had no hope of recovery (for four years). In agreement with parents, the hospital trust applied for a declaration to allow it to lawfully discontinue life-sustaining treatment and life support. The official solicitor appealed against the Court of Appeal order permitting it.

Held (House of Lords)

Removal of life support is permitted as it did not amount to murder. The actus reus of actively causing death would not be present (see Chapter 4).

Lord Goff

'The law draws a crucial distinction between cases in which a doctor decides not to provide, or to continue to provide, for his patient treatment or care which could or might prolong his life, and those in which he decides, for example by administering a lethal drug, actively to bring his patient's life to an end'.

'So to act is to cross the Rubicon which runs between on the one hand the care of the living patient and on the other hand euthanasia—actively causing his death to avoid or to end his suffering. Euthanasia is not lawful at common law'.

There was no duty to act either as treatment was not in the best interest of patient, with no prospect of recovery.

Nevertheless, in the absence of informed consent, PVS cases, or cases where patients may be in a coma, or where life-sustaining treatment has been withdrawn, as in the Tony Bland case, may be justified. On withdrawal of treatment, it is possible that there may be an agreement (between patients' next of kin and clinicians) that there is no issue. However, problems arise where there is disagreement.

Thinking Point

1   How do you establish the wishes of a patient in a PVS?
2   Did the court go too far in allowing withdrawal of treatment?

The same principle was followed and applied in the Archie Battersby case (2022). Archie, 12, had suffered traumatic brain injuries at home in Southend, Essex, on 7 April 2022. The family took the hospital trust to court and challenged as far as the Appeal Court and appealed to the UN Rights of Persons with Disabilities Committee; however, the court refused to wait for this appeal and ruled in favour of the hospital (BBC, 2022).

Case Study: Indi Gregory – Best Interests

Indi Gregory was born in February 2023, with mitochondrial disease, a genetic condition.

Indi's parents unsuccessfully fought to overturn rulings by UK High and Appeal courts to keep their daughter on life support. The appeal to the ECHR failed on the grounds that it was not in the child's best interest to travel to Rome for treatment.

(https://news.sky.com/story/indi-gregory-critically-ill-eight-month-old-baby-granted-italian-citizenship-as-uk-court-dismisses-life-support-appeal-bid-13001982)

In the recent case of Indi Gregory, a baby with mitochondrial disease, the court ruled that life support should be discontinued on the grounds that treatment would be pointless...

There may however be cases when a patient wishes to terminate their life due to a PSV, contrary to the section 2, the right to life, Article 2 of the ECHR (1950a). This is in direct contrast to Article 8, of the same statute, which defines the right to choose. It is also possible that people with unbearable conditions may feel that they are a burden to their families.

It may be challenging for loved ones and clinicians working with the patient (when the latter may feel like a 'burden'), as they aim to find the right balance in decision-making. Gudat et al. (2019) found that often terminal patients may reject external help due to privacy and aim to preserve their own dignity, as they see it, for their own 'integrity and self-control'. John Stuart Mill (1859) argued that in matters that do not affect others, individuals have the autonomy to terminate their own lives.

The principle of autonomy was tested in the Diane Pretty (2001) case below. Euthanasia or physician-assisted suicide is illegal in the UK; subject to the Suicide Act 1961, this would be 'aiding and abetting' suicide, which is illegal.

Case Law: *(R) on Application Diane Pretty v DPP [2001] UKHL 61*

Diane Pretty had motor neuron disease (MND). She wanted to control the time and manner of her death. Because of her condition, she needed help from her husband to die. She asked the government to guarantee that her husband would not be prosecuted if he helped her die.

The House of Lords rejected Diane's case on the basis that the right to life did not include a right to die. They also said that the right to private life did not include a right to decide when and how to die.

Diane took her case to the European Court of Human Rights. She argued that the right to life included a right to choose whether to carry on living. The court disagreed. They said that right to life was not determined by quality of life so could not be interpreted as also giving a right to die.

Unlike the House of Lords, they did say that Diane's right to choose how to end her life came within her right to respect for private life. But they said that the ban on assisted suicide in the UK could be justified to protect vulnerable people.

(Dignity in Dying, https://www.dignityindying.org.uk/assisted-dying/the-law/diane-pretty/)

A private member's bill, Baroness Meacher's Assisted Dying Bill (2021), fell at Committee Stage and failed to make the final stages as parliament ran out of time (2022). This principle of individual right to autonomy subject to Article 8, ECHR (1950b), in *R (on application of Purdy) v DPP [2009] UKHL 45* (a woman diagnosed with multiple sclerosis) challenged her right to autonomy and whether her husband would be prosecuted for aiding and abetting if he took her to Switzerland. Although she did not win her case, it forced the Director of Public Prosecutions (DPP) to clarify the law with new guidelines. The DPP may consent to prosecute anyone who aids and abets another, now subject to section 2A, '…as amended by section 59 and Schedule 12 of the Coroners and Justice Act (2009). Prosecutors should identify the timing of '…any alleged act of encouragement or assistance that it is alleged supports the bringing of a criminal charge relating to the suicide or attempted suicide of the victim' (DPP, 2010, para 16). This means that the UK is one of the countries which do not permit assisted suicide, punishable by 14 years imprisonment [since the CJA (2009) some clarification was introduced, with a broader remit added by section 2A].

The Isle of Man becomes the first British Isles Jurisdiction to legalise (Dignity in Dying, 2023). The Scottish Parliament's own bill is at the time of writing, underway (2023).

Do not attempt cardiopulmonary resuscitation orders (DNACPR)

DNACPR orders are not new to healthcare, and decision-making is guided by patients, next of kin, loved ones and the medical team involved. It is designed to guide healthcare professionals regarding what action to take in the event cardiopulmonary resuscitation (CPR) is needed and whether CPR is appropriate if a person has a cardiac arrest. Reasons for DNACPR orders differ according to personal choice, medical grounds for whether CPR would prevent death. Irrespective of the reason, decisions are individual and usually an multidisciplinary team decision with the patient at the centre. Equally, a ReSPECT document, a personalised recommendation of processes for an individual's future clinical emergency care and treatment, may be in place, or an ADRT or 'living will'. DNACPR and ADRT are legally binding, whereas ReSPECT is not (Resuscitation Council UK, 2024).

DNACPR has raised ethical, legal and practical dilemmas since the 1960s, but a core value is that they must be person-centred, or where not possible individual welfare and best interest must guide considerations. The decision-making may involve Advocates, Power of Attorney or appropriate use of the Mental Health Act (1983) to ensure the right decisions are made for and with the right person, for the right reasons. The Care Quality Commission (2021) extensively reported 'blanket' DNACPR orders during the COVID-19 pandemic without individual assessments. These 'blanket' DNACPR orders revealed discrimination of groups of individuals with common characteristics like age or disability, prompting a governmental working group to review the processes and training, and implement a holistic person-centred end-of-life framework (Michalowski and Martin, 2022). Irrespective of legal, political and ethical dilemma, additional burdens include barriers to the conversations and the lasting impact among healthcare staff and patients' loved ones.

Islam et al. (2021) identified personal, cultural, religious, spiritual and emotional challenges universally experienced among healthcare staff in the decision-making process with individuals and families. These emotive discussions around end-of-life care planning are often stalled by perceptions, acceptance and understanding among staff and families when considering cultural and family choices around death and dying. While there is a professional responsibility of healthcare teams, emotional labour cannot be ignored. Having difficult conversation and breaking bad news can impact healthcare professionals emotionally because they are faced with the reality of their own mortality. These emotive responses, although predominantly reported as negative, in some cases can be positive for both parties. While individuals may be shocked or distressed when discussing and writing DNACPR orders, there can also be relief for all involved. Distress at the prognosis, guilt with the decision-making, but relief of an end to suffering are all reported feelings and emotions experienced by patients, relatives and healthcare staff regarding DNACPR conversations (Hartanto et al., 2023). Sadly, COVID-19 has seen more negative impacts of end-of-life care planning and DNACPR on those closest to their loved ones and healthcare teams involved in delivering such care, while making such impossible decisions.

Thinking Point

1 Have you ever broken bad news?
2 How does it feel to break bad news?
3 How does it feel to receive bad news?
4 What emotions do you feel when you hear DNACPR?

Conclusion

Difficult as it is, end-of-life decision-making is challenging and invasive, being the most important and final choices for anyone facing them. While some patients may be able to understand and make informed choices, many more may lack capacity and would consequently not be in control. Others who are advocates or the courts may be required to make decisions on their behalf. Best interest means that the patients' welfare may be assumed by such 'surrogate' decision-makers. There are national decision-making frameworks which must be followed, and they are designed to have an outcome which is in the patient's best interests. Clinical decisions must promote the patient's welfare, even if this means the focus of care changes from life-sustaining to providing comfort and dignity. At the heart of end-of-life, palliative care (or social needs assessments) must be patient-centred with ethico-legal considerations. The aim should be to 'first do no harm' for those final critical months, weeks, days or hours of life.

End-of-life care should be distinguished from palliative care, with interventional measures which are designed to maintain patient comfort, dignity and safety. UK law, as it stands, is very clear about the fact that assisted suicide, be it (an act of kindness) by a physician or loved ones or next of kin, is a crime.

References

Access to Health Records Act (1990)

Adult Support & Protection (Scotland) Act (2007)

Airedale NHS Trust v Bland [1993] AC 789

Baroness Meacher's Assisted Dying Bill (2021)

BBC(2022)ArchiBattersbycase.Availableonlineat:https://www.bbc.co.uk/news/uk-england-essex-65192705 (Accessed on 4th January 2024)

Beauchamp and Childress (2019) Principles of biomedical ethics (8th ed). Oxford: Oxford University Press

Cadogan CA, Murphy M, Boland M, Bennett K, McLean S, Hughes C (2021) Prescribing practices, patterns, and potential harms in patients receiving palliative care: A systematic scoping review. Explor Res Clin Soc Pharm, 3, 100050. Available online at: https://doi.org/10.1016/j.rcsop.2021.100050 (Accessed on 20th February 2024)

Care Act (2014)

Care Quality Commission (2021) Protect, respect, connect—Decisions about living and dying well during COVID-19. Available online at: https://www.cqc.org.uk/publications/themed-work/protect-respect-connect-decisions-about-living-dying-well-during-covid-19 (Accessed on 13th February 2024)

Care Quality Commission (2022) Issue 5: Safe management of medicines – Treatment. Available online at: https://www.cqc.org.uk/guidance-providers/learning-safety-incidents/issue-5-safe-management-medicines (Accessed on 13th February 2024)

CBC News (2023) Available online at https://www.cbc.ca/news/politics/maid-canada-report-2022-1.7009704 (Accessed on 23rd May 2024)

Clark D (2014) Two reports that shaped the history of end-of-life care in the United Kingdom. Available online at: http://endoflifestudies.academicblogs.co.uk/two-reports-that-shaped-the-history-of-end-of-life-care-in-the-united-kingdom/ (Accessed on 31st August 2023)

Data Protection Act (2018) Available online at; https://www.legislation.gov.uk/ukpga/2018/12/contents (Accessed on 23rd May 2024)

Dignity in Dying (2023) Isle of man assisted dying bill. Available online at: https://www.dignityindying.org.uk/news/isle-of-man-assisted-dying-bill-passes-with-overwhelming-support-in-victory-for-compassion/ (Accessed on 22nd December 2023)

DPP (2010) Suicide: Policy for prosecutors in respect of cases of encouraging or assisting suicide. Available online at: https://www.cps.gov.uk/legal-guidance/suicide-policy-prosecutors-respect-cases-encouraging-or-assisting-suicide (Accessed on 20th December 2023)

European Convention on Human Rights (ECHR) Article 2 (1950a)

European Convention on Human Rights (ECHR) Article 8 (1950b)

General Medical Council (2021) Good practice in prescribing and managing medicines and devices. Available online at: https://www.gmc-uk.org/professional-standards/professional-standards-for-doctors/good-practice-in-prescribing-and-managing-medicines-and-devices (Accessed on 13th February 2024)

Gregory I (2023) Withdrawal of treatment, best interests case. Available online at: https://news.sky.com/story/indi-gregory-critically-ill-eight-month-old-baby-granted-italian-citizenship-as-uk-court-dismisses-life-support-appeal-bid-13001982 (Accessed on 10th December 2023)

Gold Standards Framework (2023). Available online at: https://www.goldstandardsframework.org.uk/gsf-awards-2023 (Accessed on 10th December 2023)

Gudat H, Ohnsorge K, Streeck N, Rehmann-Sutter C (2019) How palliative care patients' feelings of being a burden to others can motivate a wish to die. Moral challenges in clinics and families. Bioethics, 33(4), 421–430

Hartanto M, Moore G, Robbins T, Suthantirakumar R, Slowther A (2023) The experiences of adult patients, families, and healthcare professionals of CPR decision-making conversations in the United Kingdom: A qualitative systematic review. Resusc Plus, 13, 1–16. Available online at: https://www.sciencedirect.com/science/article/pii/S2666520422001515 (Accessed on 22nd May 2024)

Health Records (NI) Order (1993)

Islam Z, Taylor L, Faull C (2021) Thinking ahead in advanced illness: Exploring clinicians' perspectives on discussing resuscitation with patients and families from ethnic minority communities. Future Healthc J, 8(3), E.619–E.624

Kant E (1724–1804) Encyclopaedia Britannica (no date) Immanuel Kant | Biography, Philosophy, Books, & Facts | Britannica (Accessed on 2nd February 2024)

Marie Curie (2022a) 'What is end of life care?' Available online at: https://www.mariecurie.org.uk/help/support/terminal-illness/preparing/end-of-life-care (Accessed on 31st August 2023)

Marie Curie (2022b) 'What is palliative care?' Available online at: https://www.mariecurie.org.uk/help/support/diagnosed/recent-diagnosis/palliative-care-end-of-life-care (Accessed on 31st August 2023)

Marie Curie Memorial Foundation, Queen's Institute of District Nursing (Great Britain) (1952) Report on a national survey concerning patients with cancer nursed at home. London, Edinburgh: Marie Curie Memorial

Mental Health Act (1983)

Mental Capacity Act (2005)

Michalowski S, Martin W (2022) DNACPR decisions: Aligning law, guidance, and practice. Med Law Rev, 30(3), 434–456. Available online at: https://doi.org/10.1093/medlaw/fwac007

Mill JS (1806–1873)

National Institute for Health and Care Excellence (2015) Medicines optimisation: The safe and effective use of medicines to enable the best p[possible outcomes. Available online at: https://www.nice.org.uk/guidance/ng5 (Accessed on 13th February 2024)

National Palliative and End-of-Life Care Partnership (2021) Ambitions for palliative and end of life care: A national framework for local action 2021–2026. Available online at: https://www.england.nhs.uk/eolc/ambitions/ (Accessed on 27th November 2023)

NHS (1948) https://www.england.nhs.uk/nhsbirthday/about-the-nhs-birthday/nhs-history/

NHS (2019) The NHS long term plan. Available online at: https://www.longtermplan.nhs.uk/online-version/ (Accessed on 27th November 2023)

NHS (2023) Palliative and end of life care. Available online at: https://www.england.nhs.uk/eolc/ (Accessed on 1st March 2024)

NHS Constitution (2013)

Philp M (2015) On liberty, utilitarianism and other essays 2/e (Oxford World's Classics). Oxford: Oxford University Press

Pretty v United Kingdom 2346/02 (2002) ECHR 427 European Court of Human Rights

Public Health Oregon (2017) Oregon death with dignity act data summary 2016. Available online at: https://www.oregon.gov/oha/ph/providerpartnerresources/evaluationresearch/deathwithdignityact/documents/year19.pdf (Accessed on 10th December 2023)

R (on application of Purdy) v DPP [2009] UKHL 45

Re C (Adult, refusal of treatment) [1994] 1 All ER 819

Robson M (2021) Who the hell is Immanuel Kant? And what are his theories all about? Whothehellis.co.uk

Resuscitation Council UK (2024)

Royal Pharmaceutical Society (2019) Professional guidance on the administration of medicines in healthcare settings. Available online at: https://www.rpharms.com/publications/member-resources#AZ (Accessed on 13th February 2024)

s.2A and s59+ Schedule 12 of the Coroners and Justice (CJA) Act (2009) Available online at: https://www.legislation.gov.uk/ukpga/2009/25/section/59 (Accessed on 23rd May 2024)

S3 Suicide Act (1961) Available online at: https://www.legislation.gov.uk/ukpga/Eliz2/9-10/60 (Accessed on 22nd May 2024)

Thomas Aquinas (1225–1274) Available online at: https://www.britannica.com/biography/Saint-Thomas-Aquinas (Accessed on 23rd May 2024)

World Health Organization (2020) Palliative care. Available online at: https://www.who.int/news-room/fact-sheets/detail/palliative-care (Accessed on 31st August 2023)

Index

Printed and bound by CPI Group (UK) Ltd, Croydon, CR0 4YY

20/08/2024

01027573-0016